THE LITTLE

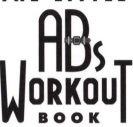

ABs WORKOUT BOOK

THE LITTLE

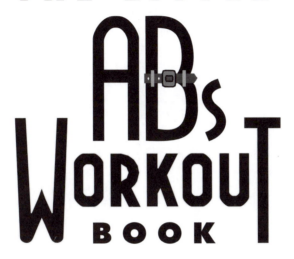

ABs WORKOUT BOOK

ERIKA DILLMAN

WARNER BOOKS

An AOL Time Warner Company

Neither these exercises and programs nor any other exercise program should be followed without first consulting a health care professional. If you have any special conditions requiring attention, you should consult with your health care professional regularly regarding possible modifications of the program contained in this book.

Warner Books, Inc., 1271 Avenue of the Americas, New York, NY 10020

Visit our Web site at www.twbookmark.com.

 An AOL Time Warner Company

Printed in the United States of America

First Printing: January 2003

10 9 8 7 6 5 4 3 2 1

Library of Congress Cataloging-in-Publication Data

Dillman, Erika.
    The little abs workout book / Erika Dillman.
       p. cm.
    Includes index.
    ISBN 0-446-67958-5
    Abdominal exercises. I. Title.

GV508.D55 2003
613.7'I—dc21   2002071343

Book design and text composition by L&G McRee
Text illustrations by Jim Chow
Cover design by Rachel McClain

For Jack

Acknowledgments

Big thanks go to everyone involved with this book: My agent, Anne Depue, my editor, Diana Baroni, assistant editor, Molly Chehak, and my friends and family for their continued support and enthusiasm.

Erin Hoover Barnett and Debby Heath for their editorial suggestions. Jim Chow for his wonderful illustrations.

And the many fitness experts who generously shared their time and expertise with me: John P. Porcari, Ph.D., Professor, Department of Exercise and Sports Science, University of Wisconsin–La Crosse; Miriam E. Nelson, Ph.D., Director, Center for Physical Activity and Nutrition, Gerald J. and Dorothy R. Friedman School of Nutrition Science and Policy, Tufts University; C. C. Cunningham, M.S., certified athletic trainer (ATC), certified strength and conditioning specialist (CSCS),

ACKNOWLEDGMENTS

ACE certified personal trainer; Darcy Norman, physical therapist, certified athletic trainer, certified strength and conditioning specialist (CSCS), Olympic Physical Therapy; Peter Cannon, personal trainer, C.H.E.K. II & Golf biomechanics C.P.F.T.; Anne-Marie Trombold, physical therapist, Performance Rehab; Sarah Scott, President, Cofounder, Ironsmith-The Fitness Doctors, U.S.A. Triathlon Coach; Phil Sanchez, B.S., ACE, ACSM Certified, Group Exercise and Pilates Director, Pacific Athletic Club, San Diego; and Michael Porter, M.S., CSCS, ACSM H/FD Certified Regional Director of Health & Fitness Education, Western Athletic Clubs, Seattle Region.

Contents

CONTENTS

Welcome to *The Little Abs Workout Book*

ABSOLUTELY ABS

It used to be that unless you were a professional bodybuilder, the state of your abs wasn't a primary concern. Today, it's all about abs. Our culture has become so obsessed with having great-looking abs that we spend millions, if not billions, of dollars every year on machines, videos, gadgets like electronic massage belts, and even "specially formulated" creams that promise to give us rock-hard abs in only eight minutes a day!

Abs have become a touchstone of fashion that reflects our standards of physical beauty, power, and attraction. Even clothes are designed to highlight the abs. It's not enough anymore to admire dreamy Calvin Klein underwear models with sweat-glistening washboard stomachs; we want to have stomachs like those.

Hollywood only perpetuates abs mania. Today's leading men and ladies can't just get by on looks or charm; they have to be buff. Even rock stars (who are supposed to be unhealthy) have transformed their images by transforming their bodies. Springsteen went from a scrawny, shaggy-headed sloucher to a bona fide hunk who could fill out a pair of Levis and a white T-shirt like, well, a Calvin Klein model. Madonna, who started off draped in lace and wearing her underwear on top of her clothes, now has abs of steel and the distinction of being named 2001 Sportswoman of the Year by *Sports Illustrated for Women* magazine.

WHAT ABOUT ME?

With all the attention focused on abs, you might be looking down at your stomach and feeling a bit intimidated. Maybe you're thinking to yourself, "That's fine for them, but what about me? Why should I care about having great abs? And what do normal people, who can't afford on-call personal trainers or devote four hours a day to exercise, do about their abs?"

Not to worry, *The Little Abs Workout Book* was written for regular people (like you and me) who want to feel and look better without spending hours in the gym or practicing dozens of repetitions of painful exercises. In this book, you'll learn how to train your abdominal and back muscles effectively to achieve the strong, flat stomach you desire.

Whether you're an absolute beginner or a frequent exerciser, you'll find exercises appropriate to your fitness level in this book.

FASHION VERSUS FUNCTION

What makes *The Little Abs Workout Book* different from so many abs books is its focus on function. Killer abs may be fashionable, but there's more to abdominal training than appearance. If you want your body to hold up to the stresses of everyday life, including your recreational and athletic pursuits, your abs need to be in top shape.

The safest, most effective way to train the abs includes a

method called "core stabilization training." The goal of this type of training is restoring optimal functioning to core (i.e., abs and back) muscles, beginning with the deepest layers of abdominal muscles that are responsible for spinal stabilization so that they can perform their designated jobs, supporting and protecting the spine.

The focus of abs training has shifted from exercises like crunches that build up the most superficial layers of the abdominal muscles (to achieve that six-pack look) to stabilization exercises that restore alignment and to functional abdominal exercises that duplicate actual movements made during daily life.

This approach may not sound as sexy as jumping into the six-pack regimen, but here's the payoff. Strong abs improve your posture, balance, and alignment, helping you sit, stand, and walk with more grace and efficiency. Strengthening abs and back muscles can also increase your energy and endurance and help reduce your risk of lower back pain. You will still get a better-looking stomach; you just need to take the time to lay the foundation first.

If, like many people, you spend your days sitting in front of a computer or behind the wheel of a car, you'll appreciate the benefits of having stronger abs. Considering that 80 percent of adults will experience lower back pain in their lives, abdominal training is a practical tool to prevent injury and improve health.

How to Use This Book

You don't have to be a trained athlete or a crop-topped rock star to benefit from having stronger, more functional abdominal muscles. Whether you're twenty-five or sixty-five, you can improve the condition of your abs.

The goal of *The Little Abs Workout Book* is to educate readers about the importance of and the techniques for training the abdominal muscles from the deepest layer to the most superficial layer, or from the inside out. There is no quick fix to getting great abs, but with patience, consistency, and dedication, you will make progress.

Those of you who hate crunches, as I do, will be happy to hear that you can achieve a taut torso without doing crunches (this book is virtually crunch-free). And for those who want that "six-pack" look, once you've restored the functionality of your abs, you can progress to exercises that focus on bulking up the superficial ab layers.

This book is based on progression, each chapter building on information presented in the previous chapter. So, in order to get the most out of this information, read the chapters in order so that by the time you reach the exercises, you have a basic understanding of the anatomy of the area, posture and alignment, and the basic philosophy and guidelines of abs training.

EMBRACE THE CHALLENGE

The Little Abs Workout Book is not about whipping yourself into shape, but about learning how to train your abs safely and effectively to achieve a stronger, more attractive body. The step-by-step program in this book was designed to help you gain a greater awareness of your body as you progress through the different phases of training.

I worked with several certified athletic and personal trainers and licensed physical therapists to select the exercises and order the progression of exercises presented in Chapters 6–11. The training begins with simple, subtle movements before introducing you to more challenging exercises.

Welcome to *The Little Abs Workout Book*

Please keep in mind that abs training is just one element of physical fitness. Exercising regularly, developing overall strength and flexibility, and eating a healthy diet are essential for best results.

Good luck, and have fun.

ERIKA DILLMAN

1 | From Flabby to Fab

AWE-INSPIRING ABS

I was blissfully unaware of my abdominal muscles until I saw Brandi Chastain rip off her shirt in jubilation after scoring the winning goal for the U.S. Women's Soccer Team in the 1999 Women's World Cup, revealing a torso so taut you could bounce a quarter off it.

Suddenly I felt weak, small, and inadequate . . . and more than a little bit jealous. There I was lounging on the couch, potato chip crumbs covering my torso, and there she was, in all her power and glory, putting women's sports on the map and forever changing the way people think about women's bodies.

In the following weeks, the press hailed Chastain and her team-mates for their chiseled bodies as much as for the skill and tenacity that led them to their World Cup victory.

INDIFFERENT ABS

I really had never noticed my abs before because I'd always been tall, thin, and in great shape (or so I thought). As a competitive runner from the age of eleven through twenty-one, I had a powerful set of lungs, a resting heart rate approximating the speed limit on the quiet streets of the small town where I grew up, strong legs, and a flat stomach. I ate whatever I wanted and didn't gain weight.

But then injuries and chronic illness forced me to drastically reduce my physical activities, and unhealthy habits like working at a computer day after day (and binging on chips) had taken their toll on my body. It had been fourteen years since my last race, and my formerly rigorous fitness regimen had dwindled down to short daily walks. My posture was awful, and my back, neck, and arms hurt. I felt like I had the body of someone my grandmother's age.

As for my abs . . . I assumed that because my stomach was still relatively flat (especially when I was lying on my back) I had good abs. But the more I thought about it, the more my denial turned to desperation. *I* wanted a great-looking stomach.

ABS EDUCATION

I became obsessed with my abs, although for the next two years I didn't do much about them but inspect myself in the mirror every day, hoping for a change.

It's not as if I hadn't been told. Over the years, my physical therapists, massage therapists, and yoga teachers had encouraged me to strengthen my abs and back muscles to improve my posture and correct muscle imbalances and weaknesses throughout my body. But what was I to do? I hated doing crunches; they hurt my neck.

In the end it wasn't only vanity that inspired me to meet with a physical therapist and a personal trainer about my abs. I was also seeking relief from constant lower back pain. I don't know why it was different this time, but I made a decision to stick with an abs plan. Maybe it was because for the first time I really made the connection between the state of my abdominal muscles and the health of my back. Plus, I just didn't want to walk around all hunched over anymore.

MY ABS PROGRAM

I started off with a few basic abdominal and postural exercises that helped me establish correct spinal alignment and learn how to contract my abdominal muscles to support that alignment. These preliminary exercises consisted of relatively simple movements, but they were surprisingly challenging (more mentally than physically).

In order to perform each exercise correctly, I had to concentrate on feeling and controlling the deepest layer of my abdominal muscles during each movement. Building endurance and coordination took time and practice.

I progressed fairly quickly, though, and gradually improved and moved on to a greater variety of exercises. I was thrilled to learn that I didn't have to do one crunch to get better-looking abs; I had choices. With the help of my trainer, I discovered many exercises that worked the abs in a variety of positions: sitting, standing, lying down, and even using a large stability ball or a medicine ball. After spending a lifetime participating in sports that required me to move as fast as possible from A to B, it was exciting to learn that I could get in shape just staying in one place, and I had fun trying to master the different exercises.

The most difficult aspect of abdominal training for me wasn't performing the exercises but having the discipline to do them almost every day. I found that if I included them near the end of my daily yoga practices I was more likely to do them.

After about a month, I started to notice some definition on the sides of my stomach, and after another month, I noticed that my love handles were getting smaller. My stomach felt firm when I pressed against it with my fingers, and I found that I was able to sit at my computer longer than I previously could before becoming fatigued.

I'd still like to increase the intensity of my aerobic activity and lose a few pounds, but I'm enjoying my abs exercises and seeing the results of maintaining my new torso. I'm happy to be feeling stronger and walking taller these days.

2 | Anatomy and Physiology

BASIC ANATOMY

The first step in abs training is understanding the anatomy and physiology of the abdominal and back muscles. Learning more about the location and function of these muscles will help you perform your abdominal exercises with greater awareness.

While performing the various exercises described in later chapters, you'll need to be able to locate, isolate, and engage specific muscles, as well as maintain muscular control and correct posture. Visualizing the muscles you're trying to train will help you perform the exercises safely and efficiently and establish a mind-body connection that will help restore healthy movement patterns in core muscles and throughout the body.

THE ABS

The abdominal muscles consist of four muscles located between the pelvis and the rib cage:

- the transverse abdominis
- the internal obliques
- the external obliques
- the rectus abdominis

Each muscle works singularly and in combination to support the spine, compress the abdomen, and move the torso. The abdominal muscles are also involved in breathing. (*See Figures 2.1 to 2.4, page 16.*)

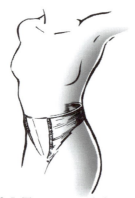

Figure 2.1 Transverse abdominis

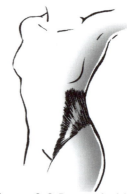

Figure 2.2 Internal obliques

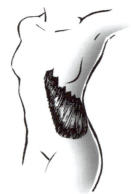

Figure 2.3 External obliques

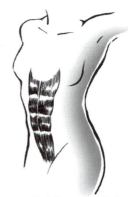

Figure 2.4 Rectus abdominis

Transverse Abdominis: The Stability Muscle

The transverse abdominis is the first layer of the abdominal muscles. Its fibers run horizontally, between the pelvis and the rib cage, wrapping around the body like a corset. You've probably heard people talk about "sucking or pulling in their guts" when referring to trying to flatten their stomachs. This action is performed by the transverse abdominis.

Stop for a minute now, and place your hands around the sides of your body (at your pelvis). Flatten your stomach by gently pulling in your gut and feel the transverse abdominis contract, reducing the diameter of your torso in that area.[1] This simple exercise also demonstrates the involvement of the abs in respiration, particularly exhalation.

The primary function of the transverse abdominis is supporting the lumbar spine (lower back) and the body's vital organs. (*See Figure 3.1, page 31.*) This job is critical to maintaining correct posture and initiating safe and efficient movements in all daily and recreational activities. When this muscle is healthy and toned, it functions automatically, but often injury, illness, inactivity, poor posture, and other habits can lead to muscle imbalances and weaknesses in the body, all of which affect the transverse abdominis.

The transverse abdominis is often overlooked in many fitness books, but it is the cornerstone of restoring function, and building balanced strength, endurance, and muscular control, in the abs. You'll read more about the transverse abdominis and its role in spinal stabilization in later chapters.

The Obliques: Internal and External

The next layer of abdominal muscles, the internal obliques, lies on each side of the torso, between the pelvis and the ribs. The muscle fibers of the internal obliques run up from the pelvis, fanning out diagonally to the ribs.

The external obliques, also located between the pelvis and ribs along the sides of the torso, make up the third layer of the abdominal muscles. They lie on top of the internal obliques, and their fibers run down from the ribs, fanning out diagonally to the pelvis.

The primary functions of the internal and external obliques are to rotate (twist) the torso, bend the torso to the side, and assist with forward flexion (bending) of the torso. They also help the transverse abdominis compress the abdomen.

To feel your obliques, grasp the sides of your torso just

below your waist with your fingers resting on the front of your body. Gently perform a side bend to your right until you feel the obliques contract in your left side. This can be done in a standing or seated position. Come back to your starting position, and this time, gently twist to the left, then to the right, feeling the obliques on both sides activate with each twist.

Next, place your hands around the sides of your body (at your pelvis), and cough. Once again, you'll feel the transverse abdominis contract. (This is a subtle movement; you should be able to maintain your normal breathing pattern.)

Rectus Abdominis: The Six-Pack Muscle

Of all the abdominal muscles, you're probably most familiar with the rectus abdominis, the muscle people refer to when they talk about six-pack abs or washboard stomachs.

The rectus abdominis is the most superficial layer of the abdominal muscles, running vertically from the front of the pelvis to the sternum (breast bone) and ribs. Its primary function is forward flexion (bending) of the torso. Like the obliques, it also helps compress the abdomen.

Many people mistakenly believe that exercising the rectus abdominis is all they need to do to get great abs. While it's true that a toned rectus abdominis can change the appearance of your stomach, the underlying muscle layers must also be toned if you want the top layer of muscle to be flat. For most people, achieving a chiseled torso also involves losing the layers of fat covering the abdomen.

In terms of function, the deeper layers of the abdominal muscles must be toned so that the abdominal muscles work together to support the spine (which, in turn, helps reduce the risk of lower back injury).

THE PELVIC FLOOR

In addition to these four commonly discussed abdominal muscles, there are several smaller muscles in the abdominal cavity that are affected by abdominal training. These muscles are located in the pelvic floor.

The pelvic floor consists of tissues, including muscles, that run from the pubic bone to the coccyx (tailbone). If you think of the lower part of your torso as a large bowl, the pelvic floor would lie against the bottom of the bowl.

Anatomy and Physiology

The pelvic diaphragm is the largest muscle group of the pelvic floor. These muscles are responsible for most of the pelvic floor's functions, including sexual function, continence, and supporting vital organs. Like other muscles in the body, the pelvic diaphragm muscles require regular exercise and can be trained to function more effectively.[2]

Strenuous exercise, pregnancy and childbirth, and other factors can weaken or injure pelvic floor muscles, commonly causing incontinence. Abdominal training, as well as Kegel exercises, strengthen the pelvic floor muscles, restoring function to the area. (To perform a Kegel exercise, squeeze your pelvic floor muscles, as if you're trying to stop the flow of urine midstream. Practicing Kegels several times a day for a few minutes at a time will help strengthen pelvic floor muscles. Check with your doctor for more detailed information on how and why to do Kegel exercises.)

There's an added bonus to having strong pelvic floor muscles: better sex. Stronger pelvic floor muscles help women achieve orgasms and help men achieve and maintain erections.

HIP FLEXORS

Hip flexors are not abdominal muscles, but it's important to understand their location and function so that you can perform abdominal exercises correctly. A common mistake made in abdominal exercises like the crunch (or sit-up) is to rely on the hip flexors rather than the abdominal muscles to help raise the torso from the floor.

The hip flexors consist of two muscles in the pelvic region, the psoas, which runs from the lumbar spine through the pelvis to the femur (thigh bone), and the iliacus, which runs from the crest of the pelvis to the femur. Both muscles are responsible for hip flexion (lifting the legs), and the psoas, along with other muscles, has the secondary function of straightening the lumbar spine.[3]

To feel your hip flexors, sit in a chair and place your fingers at the tops of your thighs, where they meet the torso. Slowly and gently raise one foot off the floor a few inches, and you'll feel a tough band of muscles contract. Those are your hip flexors.

In many of the abdominal exercises in this book, you'll be isolating your abdominal muscles so that you don't rely on your hip flexors to initiate or maintain movement. You'll notice in other exercises that your hip flexors will become engaged, but your primary mover in all of the exercises should be your abdominal muscles.

BACK MUSCLES

Muscle groups work in pairs, so when training abdominal muscles, you must also train the complementary back muscles to achieve balanced strength and endurance in the torso.

Together with the abdominals, a group of back muscles called the erector spinae, which run vertically along the spine, also assist in stabilizing the spine and moving the torso. These muscles run from the pelvis to the thoracic spine (midback), with virtually no attachment to the vertebrae in the lumbar region (lower back) of the spine. These muscles help extend the back in movements like bending or lifting. (*See Figure 2.5, page 24.*)

Another muscle group, called the multifidi, also runs along the spine. These small muscles are located deep in the back and help stabilize the lumbar spine during bending and rotation.

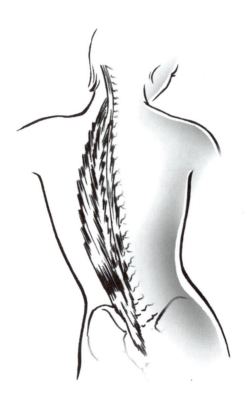

When training these muscles, you'll feel a tightening sensation along each side of your spine in the area between your ribs and pelvis. A great exercise for strengthening both the erector spinae and the multifidi is the Alternate Arm and Leg Extension on page 126.

While you can feel the erector spinae stretch as you bend forward and contract as you return to full height (you can also feel the muscles with your hand while bending forward), it takes a skilled trainer or physical therapist to locate and feel the multifidi during contraction. A more helpful cue would be to visualize that as you perform exercises, when you pull your transverse abdominis up and in toward your spine, your tailbone rises to meet the muscles (without moving your spine) to help activate the multifidi.

This concept may seem a bit confusing now, but try not to think about it too much. If you follow the instructions closely as you practice the exercises in this book, you'll gradually begin to develop a greater intuition about your movements and technique and gain the benefits of your abs workouts.

The quadratus lumborum is another back muscle you'll use during some of the abdominal exercises in this book. It's located deep in the lower back and runs between the top crest of the pelvis and the twelfth rib, on each side of the body. (*See Figure 2.6*).

The quadratus lumborum has two primary functions, side bending of the lumbar spine and ribcage and raising one hip higher than the other.[4] You'll feel the quadratus lumborum activate when practicing the Quad Burner, on page 162.

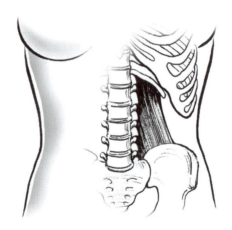

Figure 2.6 Quadratus lumborum

PUTTING IT ALL TOGETHER: THE CORE

Now that you have a basic understanding of the abdominal and back muscles and how they function, you're ready to learn how they work together to provide a strong, stable torso and how that strength and stability translates into a healthier, better-toned, more efficient, less injury-prone body.

You've probably heard or seen the term "the core" or "core training" mentioned at your health club or in fitness magazines. It's also a key concept of Pilates, an exercise method designed to strengthen the torso. Fitness professionals may vary in how they describe "the core," and even in which muscles they consider part of the core. Here, the term applies to the muscles located in the torso that are responsible for stability, endurance, movement, and strength. In other words, the abdominal and back muscles.

3 | What Are Great Abs?

FASHION AND FUNCTION

For most of us, there isn't much of a distinction between great abs and great-looking abs. If you have a washboard stomach, you have great abs. Right?

Unfortunately, this concept isn't always true because it's possible to have a flat stomach and still have a weak core. Performing endless repetitions of traditional abs exercises like sit-ups or crunches that work the superficial layer of the abs, the rectus abdominis, can produce the desired look in many people, but that approach is not the most effective at building the overall core strength that helps us move with grace and efficiency, maintain our balance and posture, and protect the lower back from injuries.

The best personal trainers know what physical therapists have taught their patients for a long time: successful abdominal training must include exercises that restore optimal functioning to the deepest layers of abdominal and back muscles that support and protect the spine.

Improving the functionality of core muscles is not only the best way to restore strength, endurance, and control to abdominal and back muscles, it's the best way to get a toned midsection.

ABS AND ALIGNMENT

The spine has three natural curves: the cervical curve, a slight forward curve at the top of the spine; the thoracic curve, a slight backward curve in the upper back; and the lumbar curve, a slight forward curve at the lower back. (*See Figure 3.1, page 31.*) In order to maintain optimal spinal alignment and posture, the abdominal and back muscles must work efficiently together.

If one muscle group is weak, or if both are, muscle imbalances occur that affect the entire body.

If you look at Figure 3.4, you'll see an example of poor posture. Her lower back is swayed, her upper back is hunched, and her head juts out in front of her body. Because her core muscles are not functioning optimally, other muscles are trying to fill in and maintain posture. This imbalance strains muscles, ligaments, and joints, and can cause lower and midback pain, neck pain, and fatigue. Poor posture can also affect the internal organs and breathing. (*See Figures 3.2 to 3.4, page 32.*)

When you add the strain and stress of working at a computer all day or a strenuous tennis match after work to a body that's already out of alignment, you risk further injury. And like it or not, our physical appearance can say a lot about our character, personality, and state of mind. Whether you're meeting friends for lunch, attending a job interview, or meeting your future in-laws for the first time, entering a room standing tall and walking gracefully makes a much better first impression than shuffling in all hunched over like a little anchovy.[1]

When core muscles are strong, they form a corsetlike support that helps maintain alignment while sitting, standing, running, or playing sports. Correct alignment helps us move more effi-

Figure 3.1 Spine

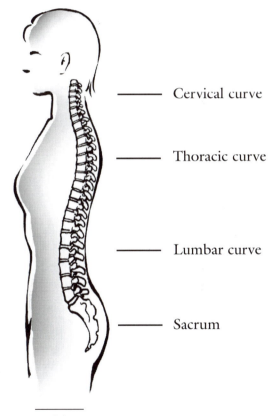

Cervical curve

Thoracic curve

Lumbar curve

Sacrum

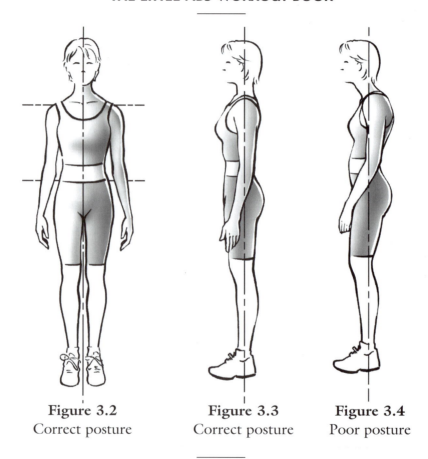

Figure 3.2
Correct posture

Figure 3.3
Correct posture

Figure 3.4
Poor posture

ciently so that we use less energy and experience less fatigue. In addition to holding your body upright, core muscles also help you keep your balance during movement.

FIVE ELEMENTS OF GOOD POSTURE

1. Stand tall.

Imagine that there is a string running vertically through your body and out the top of your head and someone is pulling up on that string. Hold your head high, with your chin parallel to the floor.

2. Relax shoulders.

Let your shoulders relax away from your ears. They should be parallel with the floor and in line with your ears, hips, and ankles.

3. Lift chest.

Slightly lift your chest to maintain correct alignment in midback.

4. Engage abs.

Flatten your stomach and support spinal alignment in the lower back by gently engaging the transverse abdominis.

5. Stand firm.

Plant your feet firmly on the floor, keep your legs straight without locking the knees, gently engage thigh muscles.

With a strong core, Figure 3.3 stands tall, head held high. Because the appropriate muscles are maintaining alignment, you don't see signs of strain in the back or neck. Notice how her ears, shoulders, hips, knees, and ankles form a straight line. Also, notice Figure 3.2's long, straight neck and relaxed shoulders, and how the shoulders and hips are parallel with the floor.

The goal of abdominal training is to achieve this level of alignment and then maintain it during movement.

THE CENTER OF POWER

Located in the center of your body, your core is literally and figuratively the center of your power. All movement originates in the core, and many other aspects of athletic prowess, such as balance, speed, agility, force, coordination, strength, and endurance, all depend on a strong core.

In yoga and martial arts, which have both been around for centuries, if not millennia, the center of the body is considered the source of life energy. Maybe you've heard the expression "breath of fire," which refers to a yoga breathing technique designed to raise the heat (or energy) of the body from bottom to top. In the yoga tradition (as in the chakra system), the center of the body is associated with fire, heat, and power, as well as emotional qualities like self-esteem, self-respect, and willpower. The goal in yoga, as in martial arts, is to harness this energy by balancing it, creating a physical and emotional centeredness from which to move.

ABS AND THE PROS

When it comes to accessing core power, professional athletcs are way ahead of the game. Athletic trainers for men's basketball and football teams have long included core training in their teams' strength-conditioning programs. And women's teams are getting into the game, too. Members of the Women's U.S. National Soccer Team and Olympic-bound skiers and bobsledders are just a few of the female athletes whose abs training programs have been featured in national sports magazines.

The core is the body's airport terminal. Every movement passes through it. An athlete can be in excellent cardiovascular condition and have strong legs and arms, but if her core muscles aren't in optimal condition, this creates a weak link in the body's muscle chain that affects all of her movements. If core muscles don't do their job to stabilize and move the torso, then arm and leg muscles will overcompensate, trying to do a job for which they are ill-equipped. This state of muscle imbalance affects all aspects of movement and strength, and can leave an athlete susceptible to injury.

Athletes must have the core strength and endurance to perform for the entire length of a competition. If an athlete can't maintain an upright position without fatigue, how can she jump higher, throw farther, or move faster than her opponents? When the core is stable and strong, athletes have the agility and explosive power to burst out of the starting blocks, serve a tennis ball at 115 miles per hour, or slam-dunk a basketball.

YOUR EVERYDAY ABS

Spinal stability and core strength are also essential for us mere mortals. In daily life, you need strong abs and back muscles to sit at your desk and work, stand in line at the grocery store, walk gracefully across a room, run, jump, scrub the soap scum off your bathroom tiles, throw, kick, work in your garden, and lift your child out of his car seat. If your core muscles are weak, these simple activities and movements can cause pain or even injury.

THE BENEFITS OF STRONG ABS

- Improved posture
- Reduced risk of lower back pain
- More efficient and powerful movements
- Greater muscle tone in stomach and torso
- Greater strength and endurance
- Enhanced breathing
- Improved sports performance
- Improved body awareness and confidence

THE MISSING LINK

Despite the large numbers of men and women who participate in regular physical activity, such as walking, jogging, or lifting weights (with women outnumbering men), the missing link in many fitness programs is abdominal training.

One of the reasons people may neglect their abs is that they don't make the connection between the state of their abs and their overall health, especially if they feel fit. People may want six-pack abs, but unfortunately, that desire is not always enough to motivate people to take action.

Many people are intimidated or put off by the idea of working on their abs because they think abdominal training will be time-consuming, difficult, painful, or worse, embarrassing. Or maybe they imagine exercising the abs as a boring endeavor involving endless sit-ups or crunches. Others may faithfully perform their abs exercises but not gain the benefits because their technique is incorrect or because they're not doing a variety of exercises to build balanced strength.

THE NEW APPROACH TO ABS TRAINING

The good news is—training your abs is not as complicated or boring as you might imagine. Nor does it require a big time commitment. In fact, in the time it takes to listen to a few songs on the radio, you can complete an abs workout.

The physical, emotional, and health benefits of having great abs provide many compelling reasons to include abs training in your regular fitness regimen. Restoring spinal stability and functionality to abdominal (and back) muscles as part of that training is essential to your success in achieving a flat, toned stomach.

In the next chapter, you'll read more about the specific philosophies and methods of effective abdominal training that will help you get great abs.

4 | How to Get Great Abs

EFFECTIVE ABS TRAINING

Great abs are the product of correct, consistent training. As you read in Chapter 3, the goals of successful abdominal training are to restore optimal spinal alignment, retrain the deepest layer of the abdominal and back muscles to support that alignment, and improve the overall strength and functioning of core muscles.

The most effective method of achieving great abs is a combination of exercises that stabilize the spine and exercises that work the core muscles in a variety of positions or movements.

SPINAL STABILIZATION

Spinal stabilization training is the first step to restoring function to core muscles. Physical therapists refer to this process as "spinal stabilization" or "lumbar stabilization," while personal trainers and fitness instructors may call it "core stabilization." All three terms refer to the same concept: training the abdominal and back muscles to support and protect the spine. When these muscles perform their designated functions, the body can maintain correct alignment, which is essential for balance, movement, and reducing the risk of back injuries.

This type of training program is very common with physical therapists, who have used it for years to help rehabilitate patients with spinal injuries or lower back pain. Now it's becoming a popular trend in the fitness world as people become more interested in overall wellness and in pursuing more purposeful exercises and activities.

NEUTRAL SPINE

The first step of spinal stabilization is developing an awareness of spinal alignment. As you can see in Figure 3.1 on page 31, the spine has a natural curve at the lumbar region. Physical therapists use the term "neutral spine" to describe optimal spinal alignment, or the position in which the spine is best able to carry load and move most safely and efficiently. It's also the position of the lower spine when the body is in correct posture. In contrast, remember Figure 3.4 (page 32), whose spine is not optimally aligned or well-supported by core muscles, and who is, therefore, less able to move gracefully and more likely to become injured.

PRELIMINARY EXERCISES

In Chapter 6, you'll begin your abs training with several simple preliminary exercises, such as the pelvic tilt, designed to help you find your ideal spinal alignment, or neutral spine. Next, you'll practice isolating and contracting the deepest layer of the abs, the transverse abdominis, while maintaining neutral spine. The goal of these exercises is to train the muscles that stabilize the spine so that supporting optimal alignment becomes automatic.

In the next group of preliminary exercises, you'll try to maintain neutral spine and contraction of the transverse abdominis while adding the challenge of moving the limbs. These initial exercises prepare abs and back muscles to maintain spinal alignment during daily activities, sports, and recreation, and lay the foundation for all of the other core exercises you'll practice in Chapters 7–11.

STRENGTH, ENDURANCE, BALANCE, AND CONTROL

Physical therapists and scientists have researched the efficacy of spinal stabilization training in the context of treating and preventing lower back pain, a common malady. Research has shown that muscle strength alone is not the most important factor in restoring optimal health to the lower back. Muscle endurance, balanced strength between muscle groups, and muscle coordination and efficiency are all essential in restoring spinal stabilization. For this reason, a variety of abs and back exercises are used to train the core while the body is in different positions.

Abs Exercises

There are primarily three types of exercises used in this book to help you successfully tone your middle: stabilization exercises, which retrain core muscles to support the spine; functional exercises, which duplicate everyday movements and activities while challenging the abs to maintain optimal spinal alignment (protecting the spine); and what I call "six-pack exercises," traditional or commonly known abs exercises that help build up the superficial layers of the abs to achieve the desired look. All of these exercises are important in building and maintaining balanced strength, endurance, and control in core muscles.

RETRAINING MUSCLES AND NERVES

If you're like most people, despite your best intentions to lead a healthy lifestyle, you've probably at some time developed muscle imbalances and weaknesses that contribute to poor posture, prevent efficient movement, and even cause injuries such as lower back pain or neck pain. Stress, injuries, overtraining, illness, inactivity, and simply living in gravity take a great toll on our bodies and can cause physical limitations.

A big part of abs training is restoring strength, endurance, and control to weak, overworked, out-of-balance core muscles by retraining muscles *and* nerves. In a healthy, aligned body muscle-nerve connections, called *neuromuscular pathways,* are established between the brain and the muscles to recruit the designated muscles for a specific function, such as sitting up straight or throwing a ball. For example, in the split second before you move, your brain sends a message, via the nervous system, to your muscles, telling them how and when to function.

If a muscle is too fatigued (due to weakness, injury, or other causes) to perform its designated function, the nerve tells the muscle what to do, but the muscle can't respond effectively. As a result, the brain, via the nerves, recruits another muscle that is not designed for that function to fill in. This muscle over-compensates trying to do the job, and over time, an unhealthy pattern gets established in which the brain continues to recruit the wrong muscle.

Effective abdominal training re-establishes healthy patterns so that the appropriate muscles are automatically recruited for each movement. Building strength in core muscles is part of training, but there are other important aspects of muscle functioning to address. Abs exercises should also help develop automatic responses like *neuromuscular control,* which refers to the coordination or efficiency with which you move, and *proprioception,* which is your body's awareness in space.

Good neuromuscular control in abdominal and back muscles helps you move with more grace and power, and improved proprioception in core muscles helps the body fight gravity and maintain balance during all movement.

THE TRANSVERSE ABDOMINIS

Retraining the deepest layer of the abdominis muscles, the transverse abdominis, is the first step in achieving balanced core strength and the taut tummy you desire.

Ideally, the transverse abdominis, pelvic floor muscles, and the multifidus muscles in the back contract concurrently to support the spine during movement. When one or all of these muscles are weak, they don't function well alone or together, leaving the spine and other areas of the body vulnerable to injury. So, before you exercise the more superficial layers of the abs, which will help you get the look you want, you have to restore optimal functioning to these deep muscles.

Working from the deepest layer of the abs to the most superficial layers (or from the inside out) is the cornerstone of successful training. The best training programs will work both the muscles that stabilize the spine and those that move the torso. Isolating the transverse abdominis in the preliminary exercises will help retrain that muscle, and once you can locate, isolate, and control it, you can gradually begin to practice exercises that integrate other core muscles through more complex movements.

PUTTING MIND TO MUSCLE

Finally, your mind will be your biggest training tool. Visualization and concentration will help you integrate and internalize the methods presented here so that you develop greater body awareness. In turn, as you become more familiar with your own anatomy and physiology, and the gradual progression of exercises, you'll gain a greater intuitive sense of how to move your body most efficiently.

In the next chapter, you'll learn some of the basic training techniques that will prepare you for the final step, beginning your abs training.

5 | Essential Training Guidelines

YOUR ABS PROGRAM

Congratulations! Taking on a new fitness challenge is a great way to preserve and improve your health. Building a strong core is one of the best fitness goals you can have; you'll feel the payoff in every move you make.

By reading the first four chapters of *The Little Abs Workout Book* you've already taken the first step toward improving the state of your abs. Opening your mind to change and learning more about how your body works are just as vital to your success as the physical aspects of abs training.

With your new knowledge of core muscles and their functions, you're ready to learn some of the specific guidelines of effective abs training.

How Great Abs Are Made

Training consistently and effectively is the best way to get great abs. However, your abdominal training is only one part of a bigger picture, your overall health, fitness, and lifestyle habits. You read earlier that a toned stomach is not always an indication of core strength. The opposite is also true; it's possible to have great abs, but not be able to see their tone through the layers of body fat covering the stomach.

Very few people are blessed with slender bodies that show muscle tone after the slightest amount of training. The rest of us have to work at maintaining our appearance, and that usually means finding ways to burn off the fat that surrounds our midsections. This is especially difficult for women, whose bodies naturally store fat in the abdomen.

Several factors influence the appearance of your torso, including how much and how intensely you exercise, diet and lifestyle habits, and genetics. Unfortunately, it is impossible to "spot reduce." Contrary to popular belief, doing sit-ups will not burn fat from your stomach. Abs exercises will tone your muscles, but you need to do fat-burning aerobic exercises and strength training to help you get rid of your gut. For best results your abs program should complement an overall health and fitness plan that includes aerobic exercise, strength training, flexibility exercises, and a healthy diet.

Health and fitness organizations such as the American Council on Exercise, the American College of Sports Medicine, and the U.S. Department of Health have made recommendations on the types and amount of exercise considered necessary and beneficial to health. In general, these guidelines include:

- Thirty to fifty minutes of moderately paced aerobic activities such as running, walking, rowing, or biking, at least five days a week
- Strength training two or three times a week to condition all major muscle groups
- Flexibility exercises, such as stretching or yoga, every day to reduce muscle tension, improve suppleness of muscles and connective tissues, and prevent injuries
- A healthy diet low in saturated fats and high in plant-based foods

Of course, beginning exercisers will have to start with shorter, less intense workouts and gradually increase to the recommended guidelines. Don't worry if your fitness regimen doesn't match the guidelines. Exercising three times a week is a great start. Also, the recommended thirty to fifty minutes of exercise most days of the week can be accumulated throughout each day. For example, three ten-minute walks in one day can add up to your daily thirty-minute requirement. Activities such as gardening and lawn work can supplement your exercise.

For some people, just increasing the amount or intensity of their exercise programs is enough to help them lose a few pounds. Others may need to work with a physician and certified personal trainer to find the best combination of diet and exercise to ignite their body's fat-burning mechanisms.

SETTING GOALS

It will take anywhere from a few weeks to several months for you to see or feel the results of your abs training. So, in order to stay motivated, it's helpful to set goals before you begin. Maybe your ultimate goal is to have a flatter stomach, a more powerful tennis swing, or better posture. In the meantime, you need short-term goals that are realistic and attainable.

CALORIES BURNED DURING ACTIVITY

Aerobics (high-impact). 235
Aerobics (low-impact) 185
Basketball 269
Bicycling (stationary) 235
Cleaning house 118
Gardening 151
Hiking 193
In-line skating 235
Rowing (machine) 286
Running (9 min/mile) 370
Sex 50
Swimming. 202
Tennis 235
Walking (15 min/mile) 151
Weightlifting 101
Yoga 168

Figures are not exact and are provided as a guideline only. Calculations based on 140-pound person, exercising for thirty minutes. Individual figures will vary based on weight, exercise intensity, and other factors. Exercising for a longer period of time will help burn more calories.

Sources for calorie chart include www.caloriecontrol.org, www.msnbc.com, and www.global-fitness.com.

Maybe your short-term goals could be mastering some of the mental and physical techniques that will help you improve your abs. Another example of a short-term goal could be simply sticking to your abs training schedule. Be patient and kind to yourself, and give yourself credit for wanting to make a change.

Also, remember that your body is unique: Progress at your own pace and try not to compare yourself to other people. With time, dedication, and regular practice, you will see improvement. The exercises in this book are presented in a progression to help you develop a greater awareness of the small steps you'll be taking to achieve better abs.

HEALTH CONSIDERATIONS

It's always wise to consult your physician before beginning any new fitness plan, especially if you have a known health condition. Many of the exercises in this book may not be appropriate for people with certain health problems and should not be done by pregnant women. In these cases, have your doctor approve any exercises you want to do.

If you have lower back pain or a history of back or neck

problems, your doctor may also want you to see a physical therapist who can assess your muscle strength and coordination and recommend the best approach for you.

Part of training the abs effectively is training safely. Pay attention to your form, which will help you prevent injuries, and to how your body feels during exercises. Not every exercise will be appropriate for you; that's why there are more than thirty exercises to choose from in this book. If an exercise doesn't feel right, move on to the next one, and if any movements cause pain, stop immediately.

If you have further questions, or feel that you need assistance beginning your ab routine, it's worth spending the money on a couple of sessions with a qualified, certified personal trainer who can assess your strength, coordination, and technique.

Warm Up, Cool Down

Always prepare your muscles for an abs workout with a short warmup that includes five to ten minutes of light aerobic activity (such as walking, jogging, or riding a stationary bike). A good warmup increases blood flow to the muscles, preparing them for exertion. Following your warmup with a few minutes of stretching increases muscle and connective tissue flexibility, further preparing muscles for activity and reducing injury risk.

If you practice yoga, you may prefer to do a short yoga practice as part of your warmup instead of stretching. The important thing to remember is to stretch all major muscle groups, especially lower back muscles. For more information about stretching, consult a personal trainer, yoga instructor, or a book about stretching. *Stretching,* by Bob Anderson, is an excellent resource.

The exercises in this book have been organized into five workouts for simplicity, gradually increasing in difficulty. You can practice the exercises in the order they appear or in any order you like. If you find that one or two exercises in a workout don't feel right for you, you can do more sets of the other exercises in that workout or substitute exercises from another workout. Just be careful not to try any exercises that are too difficult for you.

Maintain Control and Form

In this book, "correct form" or "correct posture" refers to the spinal position you want to maintain throughout the many movements you make. (See the neutral spine exercise on page 72 and the box on good posture on page 33.) Before each exercise, you'll find neutral spine, then engage your transverse abdominis to support that position. You'll maintain this form and control of the muscle contraction throughout each exercise.

Maintaining muscle control and correct posture, or form, while performing each exercise will help retrain abs and back muscles, restoring function. Regular practice will reinforce this process. Using correct form is also vital to preventing spine or back injuries.

During your abs workout, you might find that you need to stop between exercises and stretch your lower back. The exercises in Chapters 6–11 include two back stretches that you can do whenever you feel the need to release tension in the lower back. It's also a good idea to end your workout with some light stretching.

REPS AND SETS

If you're new to exercise, you may be unfamiliar with the terms *reps* and *sets*. A rep is one repetition of an exercise. (For many of the exercises in this book, completing an exercise once on each side of the body constitutes one rep.) In order to build strength and endurance, an exercise must be repeated enough times to create fatigue in the muscles. A general guideline for building strength is 8–12 repetitions.

A set is one group of repetitions. For example, if you do 8–12 reps of an exercise, that equals one set. If you do another 8–12 reps, that is another set.

PLANNING AN ABS WORKOUT

You can start with one set of 8–12 reps, and if you want to make your workout longer or more challenging, you can gradually work up to two or three sets.

You might find that for many exercises, one set is sufficient. Some exercises will be so challenging that you might only be able to do 4 or 5 reps. Take your time, and work within your limits. You should be able to perform at least one set of each exercise using correct form before you add more sets. It is common to spend 4–5 weeks practicing a workout before adding new exercises or progressing to a new workout.

QUALITY OVER QUANTITY

To train the abs effectively, the quality of your practice is more important than the quantity. It's better to do ten repetitions of an exercise in correct form than to do one hundred repetitions in poor form. Maintaining correct form throughout the exercises is the key to retraining muscles and nerves and restoring correct posture, freedom of movement, and greater torso strength.

Control your muscles and movements through a full range of motion. In other words, use control as you initiate a movement (i.e. during the primary exertion of the exercise) and as you return to your starting position. Focus your attention on the muscles at work, and don't rely on momentum or other muscles (like the hip flexors) to move the body during exercises.

USE YOUR HEAD

Concentration and visualization are two important aspects of effective abs training that are essential to your physical success. Try to perform each exercise using slow, controlled movements while you concentrate on maintaining correct form. Visualizing the position of the spine and pelvis and the action of the muscle will help you use correct form.

ADD VARIETY

Another key to successful abs training is variety. Performing endless crunches doesn't build balanced core strength or prepare you for the many movements you make throughout the day. It only prepares you for doing more crunches. Get off your back and try some new exercises that challenge both abs and back muscles from a variety of angles. After time your muscles will get used to performing the same exercises, so you need to change your routine every four to six weeks to prevent boredom and keep muscles challenged. You can change your workout by increasing intensity, changing the order of exercises, adding new exercises or more sets, or modifying some of your favorite exercises to make them more difficult.

Train Frequently

Consistency is vital to success. For best results train your abs three to four times a week. This schedule gives you a few rest days during the week, allowing the muscles necessary recovery time. Beginners can start with two to three times a week.

Adding Ab Work to Your Fitness Routine

Abs workouts can easily be added to your existing fitness routine and only take five to ten minutes to complete. Once you've warmed up you can do your abs workout before or after a cardio workout. The important thing is to work the abs before you become too fatigued to perform the exercises correctly. On strength-training days, you might want to add your abs exercises in the middle of your strength workout.

ADAPTING ABS EXERCISES TO YOUR LEVEL

As you progress with your abs workout, you may want to make minor adjustments to specific exercises to make them more challenging. There are several simple ways to do this.

You can add weight or resistance to the move (for example, performing a basic squat while holding a medicine ball makes the core muscles work harder), use a longer lever (you can increase the challenge of doing a crunch on a stability ball by extending your arms over your head instead of placing them crossed over your chest), and introduce instability (exercises performed on stability balls and wobble boards force deep core muscles to work harder to maintain balance while performing movement). Other ways to increase the challenge include increasing the pace or intensity and adding more reps or sets.

Remember, form is critical. If you try a more challenging variation of an exercise and can't maintain correct form, you're not ready to progress to that variation yet.

BREATHING

It may seem strange, but many people forget to breathe when doing abs exercises. Holding your breath during exercise is actually harmful, so you need to practice correct breathing technique. In some exercises you'll exhale (through your mouth) when making the major move of the exercise and inhale (through the nose or mouth) when returning to the starting position. In other exercises you'll inhale with movement and exhale with release. Each exercise in this book will include breathing instructions. If you find it too difficult to coordinate your breath and movement, just breathe normally.

In addition to integrating your movements and breathing, you will be instructed to hold a position in some exercises for five, ten, or more seconds. During holds, continue to breathe normally, counting "one Mississippi, two Mississippi," etc. If you can, take slightly longer, deeper breaths (both inhaling and exhaling more slowly) to help you hold the position for a full count.

ABS MACHINES

According to the National Sporting Goods Manufacturers Association, people spent $135 million in 2000 on machines and gadgets to work their abs. You've probably seen the ads for these machines in the Sunday paper, in magazines, and on countless TV infomercials and wondered if they're worth the money.

Researchers at several U.S. universities have concluded that they aren't. The consensus about abs machines is that while most of these machines won't harm you, they aren't any more effective at training the abs than floor exercises that you can do for free.

One research study commissioned by the American Council on Exercise rated several common abs exercises for effectiveness in working both the rectus abdominis and the obliques. Top-ranked exercises included the Bicycle (see page 144), the captain's chair (not included here because it is an advanced-level exercise that can cause injury if not performed correctly, and it requires equipment only found in health clubs), and Crunch on a Ball (see page 132).

You might be surprised to learn that the crunch, the most common abs exercise, was ranked seventh in working the rectus and eleventh in working the obliques. Variations on the crunch ranked higher. (For more information, check out the American Council on Exercise's website at www.ace.org.)

Despite their findings, many researchers agree that if buying an abs machine helps someone begin or stick with an exercise program, it might be worth the expense.

However, if you're thinking of buying an abs machine, you're better off buying low-cost "props" like a stability ball ($25 to $45), a medicine ball ($15 to $20), and a wobble board ($35 to $65). All of these items are usually available for use at health clubs, and are by no means essential to abs training, but if you prefer to exercise at home, they can add fun and variety to your routine.

Stability balls, often used by physical therapists in rehabilitation training and now popular in the fitness world, are large rubber balls (forty-five to sixty-four centimeters in diameter) on which exercises can be practiced. The balls introduce instability to exercises so that the abs are forced to respond in order to maintain the balance necessary to do the exercises. Stability balls are also called exercise balls, therapy balls, or balance balls.

Medicine balls, small, weighted balls (six to eight inches in diameter) have been used by professional athletes for years to increase resistance during exercise. These simple tools are also excellent for functional training exercises.

Wobble boards are round or square wooden boards (sixteen to twenty-two inches in diameter or 16" x 16" or larger in area) with small half spheres attached to their undersides. When you stand on the board, it wobbles from side to side, and as you try to maintain your balance (and keep the board parallel to the floor), the core muscles are activated. (See pages 173–175 for equipment information.)

PROGRESS TO SUCCESS

Progression is another important element of effective abs training. The exercises in this book are presented as five separate workouts that lead you through a gradual progression of body awareness, motor skills, and strength and endurance training. Mastering the preliminary exercises is essential for establishing correct form—whether you are a beginner or a trained athlete.

Once you can perform the preliminary stabilization exercises in the next chapter with control (without losing form), you can progress to the first workout, then, as you improve your strength and technique, you can move on to the following workout until you gradually make your way to the final chapter.

6 | Exercises for a Taut Torso

BUILDING A FOUNDATION

The best way to achieve balanced core strength and a taut tummy is to train the abs as you would build a house—start with a strong foundation and build up.

When training the abs, you begin with the deepest layer, the transverse abdominis, and work up to the more superficial layers. Learning to isolate, contract, and control this muscle is the first step in changing the strength and appearance of your torso.

THE EXERCISES

The seven exercises in this chapter are stabilization exercises designed to help you retrain the deepest layer of your abdominal muscles, the transverse abdominis.

You'll start with a basic posture exercise, then learn how to isolate the transverse abdominis to support the spine. Once you have established correct posture and know how to contract the transverse abdominis to maintain that alignment you can progress to exercises that challenge and build balance, endurance, neuromuscular control, and strength in the other core muscles.

Don't be fooled by the apparent simplicity of these exercises. When performed correctly, they are actually quite challenging. Learning to isolate, activate, and control the transverse abdominis is difficult for people of all fitness levels.

TAKE YOUR TIME

Producing lasting change in the body takes patience, dedication, and time. It can take weeks, even months, for some people to master the stabilization exercises in this chapter (and sometimes even longer to see visible changes in muscle tone). Take your time with each exercise, and remember to use correct form. In addition to retraining your muscles, you'll also be training your mind to learn new techniques, recognize correct posture, and help you control your movements.

WATCH YOUR BACK

As you have read throughout this book, the abdominal muscles' primary function is supporting and protecting the spine. All of the daily activities in which we participate and all of the movements we make can put the spine at risk of injury if we don't have correct alignment. In order to maintain correct alignment, we need strength, balance, control, and endurance in core muscles.

Abs training, like many other fitness pursuits, can be strenuous. That's why mastering the stabilization exercises is a vital component in your abs training. All of these exercises will help you learn how to use correct form and how to contract your transverse abdominis to protect the spine while sitting, standing, and moving, preventing lower back injury.

With each exercise, pay attention to your form and keep your abs contracted throughout every movement. For balanced core strength, you'll also be doing back-strengthening exercises in each workout. Even if you cannot complete all of the abs exercises in a workout, make sure you include at least one back-strengthening exercise. Finally, don't forget to stop and stretch your lower back if necessary between exercises.

BEFORE YOU BEGIN

If you haven't already read the first five chapters of this book, please do so before practicing any of the exercises so that you understand the basic philosophies and techniques, as well as the health considerations, of safe and effective abs training.

HOW TO FOLLOW THE INSTRUCTIONS

For best results, read through all the exercise instructions and the tips and modifications lists to familiarize yourself with the movements you'll be making before practicing them. Then reread the instructions as you practice each exercise. Illustrations are provided to reflect the essence of the exercise, but please refer to the written instructions as your guide.

It's worth repeating: If you feel any discomfort, pain, or dizziness while exercising, stop immediately, and do not practice any exercises that your doctor considers inappropriate for you.

WHAT TO EXPECT

If you've ever done crunches or sit-ups before, you might expect to feel that burn up and down your stomach when you do abs exercises. Although you will feel that sensation in some of the later workouts that contain "six-pack" exercises, you won't feel the burn during stabilization exercises because the contraction of the transverse abdominis is a much more subtle movement (you'll feel a tightening in the lower abdomen) than contracting the top layer of the abdominal muscles, the rectus abdominis. In fact, one of your goals during these preliminary exercises is to contract the transverse abdominis without actively contracting the rectus abdominis.

EXERCISE 1: NEUTRAL SPINE

The first step in effective abs training is learning how to find neutral spine. Becoming more aware of your optimal spinal alignment will help you maintain good posture throughout your daily activities.

Instructions

1. Lie on your back with your knees bent, arms over your head, feet flat against the floor. Your feet should be a few inches apart, with heels 8–12 inches away from your buttocks. Lie still for a few minutes, breathing normally and observing the position of your lower back. You should have a small natural curve in the lower back. Place your hand in the small hollow between your back and the floor. Then return your arms to your sides.

2. Using your lower back muscles, slowly arch your lower back while maintaining contact with the floor with the rest of your body. Notice how your pelvis shifts or rolls forward.

Figure 6.1
Neutral Spine

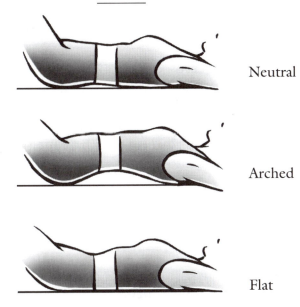

Neutral

Arched

Flat

3. Next, using your abdominal muscles, slowly press your lower back against the floor. (This movement is called a pelvic tilt.) Feel your pelvis roll backward with this movement.

4. Release the contraction of your abdominal muscles and allow your back to return to its normal, or "neutral," position. Do 1 to 3 sets of 8–12 reps.

EXERCISE II: ACTIVATING THE ABS

The next step in effective abs training is learning how to isolate and activate the deepest layer of the abdominal muscles, the transverse abdominis, to support spinal alignment. Some people call this exercise "abdominal hollowing." It's an excellent stability exercise and forms the baseline position for all the abs and back exercises to follow.

Instructions

1. Lie on your back with your knees bent, arms over your head, feet flat against the floor. Your feet should be a few inches apart, with heels 8–12 inches away from buttocks. Lie still for a few minutes, breathing normally and observing the position of your lower back. You should have a small natural curve in the lower back.

2. While maintaining neutral spine, contract your transverse abdominis, pulling it up and in toward the spine. This should be a subtle and painless movement, and the back should not

Figure 6.2 Activating the Abs

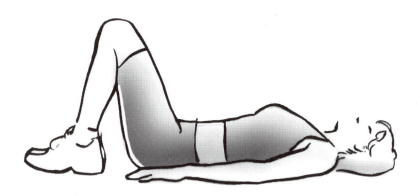

move. Visualize the sides of your pelvis moving closer together. Your rectus abdominis should remain relatively relaxed.

3. Hold this contraction for 10 seconds, breathing normally. Release. As you improve, try holding the contraction for 20 seconds, then 30 seconds, or longer. Do 1 to 3 sets of 8–12 reps.

4. Next, contract the transverse abdominis again, but this time, first pull up on your pelvic floor (as if you were trying to stop the flow of urine midstream), then pull your transverse abdominis up and in toward the spine. Visualize zipping up your muscles from your pubic area to your sternum (breastbone). Also visualize your transverse abdominis and your spine moving toward each other. This will help activate the small muscles in your back that help stabilize the spine. With practice, these small movements will become one fluid movement.

5. Hold this contraction for 10 seconds, breathing normally. Release. As you improve, try holding the contraction for 20 seconds, then 30 seconds, or longer. Do 1 to 3 sets of 8–12 reps.

Tips and Modifications

- This exercise can also be practiced in a sitting, standing, or kneeling position.
- Some fitness instructors use the expression "navel to spine" to describe transverse abdominis contraction. If you hear this in a class, remember that contracting the deepest layer of the abs is a subtle movement; your navel should move only slightly with contraction. Remember to pull up and in.
- Practice maintaining neutral spine and activating the transverse abdominis while performing daily tasks like sitting, cleaning house, driving, walking, and gardening.

EXERCISE III: ABDOMINAL BREATHING

This exercise will help you relearn correct alignment in a new position while also demonstrating the abdominal muscles' role in breathing.

Instructions

1. Kneel on the floor on all fours. Breathe normally as you find neutral spine.

2. Once you are in position, inhale slowly through your nose, filling your lungs with air. As your lungs expand, allow your belly to sink toward the floor, but maintain your neutral spinal position. Notice that your rectus abdominis is relaxed.

3. As you slowly empty your lungs, exhaling through your nose or mouth, notice how your abdominal muscles contract to help expel the air. Again, your rectus abdominis should remain relatively relaxed because the transverse abdominis is doing most of the work. Do 1 to 3 sets of 8–12 reps.

Figure 6.3 Abdominal Breathing

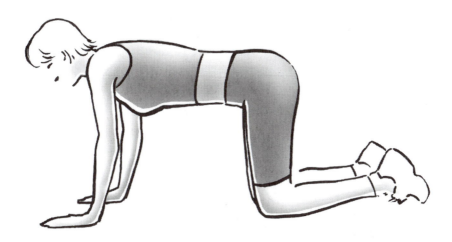

Tips and Modifications

- If you can't breathe through your nose, it's okay to breathe through your mouth.

EXERCISE IV: THE DYING BUG SERIES

This progressive series incorporates the principles learned in the previous three exercises and presents the next step in effective abs training, maintaining stable spine (spine in neutral position and transverse abdominis contracted) while introducing movement of the limbs. The Dying Bug Series has several different variations and is commonly prescribed by physical therapists and fitness trainers.

Your goal in this exercise is to maintain neutral spine throughout all the movements. You'll be using your transverse abdominis to prevent your back from arching or flattening against the floor when you move. Do not progress to the next step of the exercise until you can perform each step while maintaining correct form.

Although the Dying Bug may look simple, this series of movements is very challenging, and mastering this exercise is critical to retraining your abs to support spinal alignment during movement. Once you master this exercise, you will have established correct form and muscle control that will allow you to train safely and effectively. Do not progress to Workout One in the next chapter until you can do the Dying Bug correctly.

Instructions

1. Lie on your back with your knees bent, arms at your sides, feet flat against the floor. Your feet should be a few inches apart, with heels 8–12 inches away from buttocks. Lie still for a few minutes, breathing normally and observing the position of your lower back. You should have a small natural curve in the lower back.

2. Maintaining neutral spine, contract your transverse abdominis and the deep back muscles that run along the spine. (You may not be able to feel or control your back muscles,

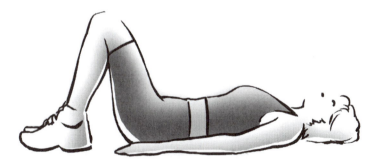

Figure 6.4 Dying Bug Series (steps 1 and 2)

but visualizing your spine and transverse abdominis moving toward each other will help activate them. You'll use this technique in all of the following steps.) Hold contraction for 10 seconds.

3. Again, in neutral spine position, contract your transverse abdominis and your deep back muscles. Slowly lift your left foot 3–4 inches off the floor. Hold this position for 5–10 seconds, then slowly lower your foot to floor. Repeat with right foot.

   If you can maintain neutral spine in this position, continue

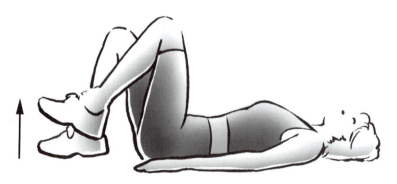

Figure 6.4 Dying Bug Series (step 3)

to the next step. If you can't, continue practicing steps 1–3 over time until you are ready to progress.

4. Contract your transverse abdominis and your deep back muscles as you straighten your left leg without touching the floor. (Your heel will be a few inches above the floor.) Hold contraction for 5–10 seconds, then slowly lower raised leg to floor. Repeat with right leg. Maintain neutral spine throughout.

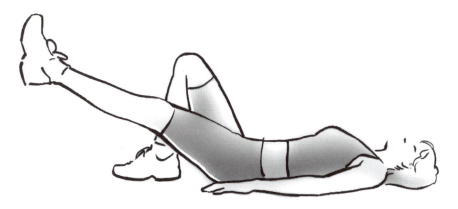

Figure 6.4 Dying Bug Series (step 4)

Figure 6.4 Dying Bug Series (step 5)

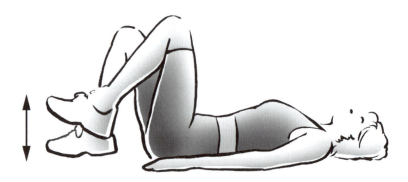

5. Contract your transverse abdominis and your deep back muscles as you slowly lift your left foot 3–4 inches off the floor. As you slowly lower it back to the floor, raise your right foot 3–4 inches off the floor. Continue alternately raising and lowering feet, gently tapping feet to floor. Continue until both feet have touched the floor 8–12 times. Then return to starting position. Maintain neutral spine throughout.

Figure 6.4 Dying Bug Series (step 6)

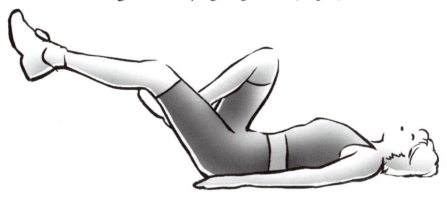

6. Contract your transverse abdominis and your deep back muscles as you straighten your left leg without touching the floor. As you bend your left leg back toward your body, extend your right leg, without touching the floor. Continue alternately moving legs in and out, as if you're pedaling a bicycle. After both legs have been extended 8–12 times, return to starting position. Maintain neutral spine throughout.

Figure 6.4 Dying Bug Series (step 7)

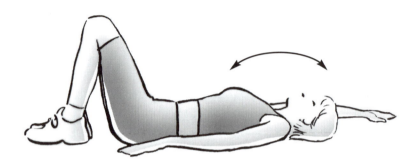

7. Contract your transverse abdominis and your deep back muscles as you lift your right arm over your head. As you return your right arm to your side, lift your left arm over your head. Continue to alternately raise and lower your arms until both arms have been extended over your head 8–12 times. Maintain neutral spine throughout.

Figure 6.4 Dying Bug Series (step 8)

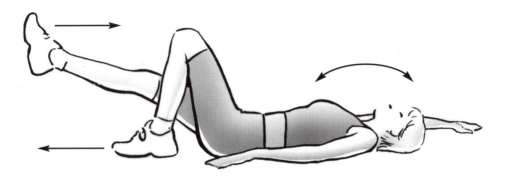

8. Contract your transverse abdominis and your deep back muscles as you slowly lift your right arm over your head at the same time you straighten and extend your right leg (without allowing leg to touch the floor). As you return your arm and leg to their original positions, slowly lift your left arm over your head and extend your left leg. Continue to alternate your arm and leg positions for 8–12 cycles. Return to starting position. Maintain neutral spine throughout. Do 1 set of 8–12 reps of each step.

Tips and Modifications

- Maintain neutral spine and constant muscle contraction.
- It's worth repeating; when the instructions say to contract your transverse abdominis and deep back muscles, you may not be able to feel your deep back muscles. Instead, visualizing that your spine and transverse abdominis are moving toward each other (without actually moving the spine) each time you contract your transverse abdominis will help activate the back muscles. If this concept is too confusing, simply focus on maintaining neutral spine and contracting the transverse abdominis.
- Increase the challenge of each movement by increasing the holding time, the number of repetitions, or the number of sets.
- Use slow, controlled movements; maintain abs contraction as you raise and as you lower arms or legs.
- Self-test: You can place your hand under the curve in your lower back to feel if your back moves up and down as you move. It should not arch up or flatten against the floor with movement, but remain in neutral position.

EXERCISE V: BACK STRENGTHENING

In order to develop balanced torso strength, you have to work the back muscles as well as the abs. This back exercise strengthens the erector spinae muscles, which are responsible for moving the torso and for holding it upright, and the multifidus muscles, which help support the spine.

Instructions

1. Kneel on the floor on all fours. Breathe normally as you find neutral spine.

2. Contract your transverse abdominis as you raise your right arm in front of you until it is parallel with the floor. Continue breathing normally while you hold this position for 5–10 seconds. Slowly release and lower your arm. Repeat with left arm (not illustrated). Maintain neutral spine and abs contraction throughout exercise and use slow, controlled movements.

3. Next, raise your left leg until it is parallel with the floor. Continue breathing normally while you hold this position for

5–10 seconds. Release and lower your leg using slow, controlled movement. Repeat with right leg (not illustrated). Maintain neutral spine and abs contraction throughout.

4. Now, contract your transverse abdominis as you raise your right arm and left leg at the same time, holding them parallel to the floor for 5–10 seconds. Slowly lower your arm and leg and repeat with left arm and right leg. Maintain neutral spine and abs contraction throughout. Do 1 to 3 sets of 8–12 reps of this step.

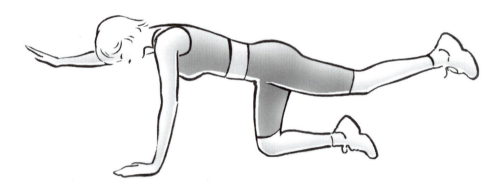

Figure 6.5 Back Strengthening

EXERCISE VI: ABS STRETCHER

If you want to stretch the front of the torso (and abs), this stretch can be done at the end of your workouts. Be careful practicing this stretch because it can compact the lower spine. Use correct form, pay attention to how your back feels, and follow this stretch with at least one set of the following back stretches to stretch the lower back.

Instructions

1. Lie on the floor in a prone position with your hands flat against the floor next to your shoulders. Before you move, press your pubic bone and hips into the floor. Maintain this contact throughout the stretch.

2. As you inhale, slowly raise your upper body off the floor. Try to maintain this position with your back muscles, so that your arms don't have to support you. If you can, extend your arms. Or keep them bent if that's more comfortable.

3. Feel the stretch in the front of your body as you extend your spine. With an exhaling breath, slowly rotate your torso to

Figure 6.6 Abs Stretcher

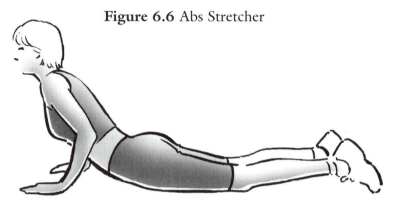

the right and hold that stretch for 10–30 seconds. As you inhale, return to center and hold that stretch for 10–30 seconds. Repeat on opposite side. Repeat 8–12 times. Follow this stretch with the Back Stretch on the next page.

Tips and Modifications

- If this stretch is too difficult, or is uncomfortable in any way, simply lie on your back, stretch your arms over your head, and reach with your fingers and toes to stretch the torso.
- Spend more time stretching if needed.

EXERCISE VII: BACK STRETCH

Now that you've completed your first abs workout, it's a good idea to end with a gentle back stretch. This stretch can be done at the end of each workout in the book, or at any time during a workout to relieve tension in the lower back.

Instructions

1. Kneel on the floor on all fours. Breathe normally as you find neutral spine. Keep your upper back and neck straight, eyes focused on a point on the floor a few feet in front of you.

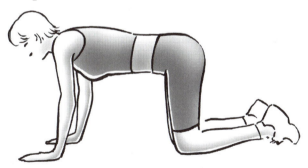

Figure 6.7 Back Stretch (step 1)

Figure 6.7 Back Stretch (step 2)

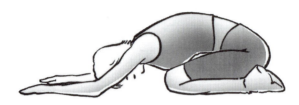

2. With an exhaling breath, use your deep abs to execute a pelvic tilt before slowly lowering your buttocks to your heels. Allow the upper back to relax and round as you lower your chest to your knees and rest your forehead on the floor.

3. As you inhale, keeping your abs engaged, raise your body back into the starting position, releasing the pelvic tilt as you return to neutral spine. Repeat stretch 8–12 times.

Tips and Modifications

- Use slow, controlled movements.
- Spend more time stretching if needed.

PROGRESSION

Once you can perform all of these exercises while maintaining correct form, you can progress to Workout One in the next chapter. As you gradually progress to each workout, remember to always warm up, and then begin each workout with the pelvic tilt and at least one stage of the Dying Bug series from this chapter. Beginning every ab workout with a few stabilization exercises will help you establish correct alignment before attempting more challenging exercises.

MANAGING YOUR WORKOUTS

As you work your way through the workouts in the following chapters, some exercises may seem easy to you and others may be very challenging. Remember that exercises will differ in how they feel in your body when you do them. In general, you'll feel a tightening across the abdomen when you do stabilization and functional exercises while holding the contraction of the transverse abdominis. During the "six-pack" exercises, like the Seated Rotation in Workout Two, you'll feel more of a burning sensation along the length of the rectus abdominis muscle. Some exercises may contain elements of both functional and "six-pack" exercises. All of the exercises will strengthen your abs and help you get a more toned stomach.

Of course, your body is unique, and what you feel in an exercise may be different from what someone else feels. If you pay attention to your body and take your time, you'll learn what each exercise will feel like for you. As a guideline, I've designated each exercise by type (stabilization, functional, six-pack, or a combination) to help you understand the various ways the abs and back muscles work during movement.

7 | Workout One: Keeping Your Balance

This group of exercises incorporates moves to challenge your balance, making core muscles work harder to stabilize the spine. Your goal, as always, is to maintain neutral spine throughout the exercises.

EXERCISE 1: SEATED ROTATION WITH A MEDICINE BALL

In the first functional exercise, you'll be using a 2- to 4-pound medicine ball to increase the challenge of a simple twisting movement. If you don't have a medicine ball, you can use a basketball or soccer ball, or even a plastic bottle filled with water. Whatever object you use, make sure that it isn't too heavy.

Instructions

1. Sit tall on the floor in good posture with legs together, extended in front of you. (If this is too difficult, you can bend your knees or place a rolled-up towel under your knees.) Breathe normally.

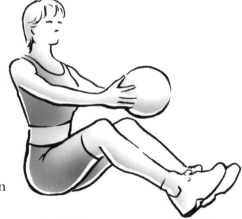

Figure 7.1
Seated Ball Rotation
(step 1)

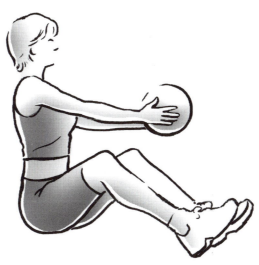

Figure 7.1 Seated Ball Rotation (step 2)

2. Maintain this posture (neutral spine) while breathing normally and holding a ball at chest level. If you can, extend your arms so that you're holding the ball away from your chest. Take slow, deep breaths into the abdomen and stay in position for up to two minutes. Next, with an exhaling breath, rotate to

the left, stopping yourself at 90°. Inhale, returning to the center. Repeat on opposite side. Do 1 to 3 sets of 8–12 reps, maintaining correct posture.

3. Optional (not illustrated): From the starting position, with the ball at your chest, lift the ball straight into the air, then lower it. Use slow, controlled movements and maintain posture. Do 1 to 3 sets of 8–12 reps.

Tips and Modifications

• To increase the challenge of this exercise, increase the pace while maintaining correct form. Or try this exercise while sitting on a stability ball.

EXERCISE II: STANDING OBLIQUE TWIST

This combination functional and "six-pack" exercise is excellent for strengthening the core and improving balance. It works all layers of the abs, as well as back muscles. The key is to keep the torso stable and relaxed and maintain your balance while moving your arms and legs.

Instructions

1. Stand in correct posture with your feet almost hips-width apart. Extend your arms from your sides, parallel to the floor and bent at 90° angles so that your hands are aligned above your elbows (and elbows aligned with shoulders).

2. With an exhaling breath, engage your transverse abdominis and rotate your torso to the left while raising your right

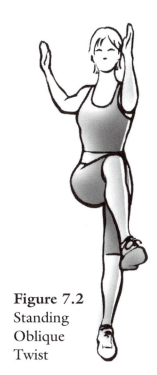

Figure 7.2
Standing
Oblique
Twist

knee (until the thigh is parallel with the floor). Your left elbow and right knee should line up, but not touch each other. Don't lift your knee too high or lower your elbow; maintain correct alignment.

3. As you inhale, rotate your torso back to the starting position, lowering leg. Repeat on opposite side. Do 1 to 3 sets of 8–12 reps.

Tips and Modifications

• It's a good idea to stretch your lower back after this exercise. Repeat Back Stretch on page 93 or Knees to Chest on page 112.

The following exercises (III-VI) help strengthen core muscles and improve balance.

EXERCISE III: BALANCE ON BALL

Using a stability ball helps train the deep layers of core muscles that support the spine. The instability of sitting on a moving ball challenges abs and back muscles to establish and maintain correct pelvic and spinal alignment. Your goal is to maintain your balance and posture.

Make sure that the stability ball you use is the correct size for your height. Each manufacturer has its own sizing charts, but in general, if you're between 5'1" and 5'7", you need a 55-cm ball, and if you're between 5'8" and 6'2", you'll need a 65-cm ball. Smaller and larger balls are available.

If you don't have a stability ball, you can practice establishing and maintaining correct posture (Exercises III–VI) while sitting in a chair, although the exercises will not be as challenging. Or you can proceed to the next workout in chapter 8.

Instructions

1. Sit in correct alignment on the top of your stability ball. Your thighs should be parallel to the floor, feet flat on floor, knees aligned over your ankles. Breathe normally.

2. Notice how the deepest layer of your abs contracts as you try to maintain your balance. The ball may move around a little bit, but try to keep it still. Staring at a point in front of you will help you focus on your balance. Maintain neutral spine. Stay on ball for several minutes if you can.

Tips and Modifications

- Use a stability ball in an open area, away from furniture, in case you roll off the ball.
- Adult-sized stability balls are not suitable for children to climb or play on.

Figure 7.3
Balance on Ball

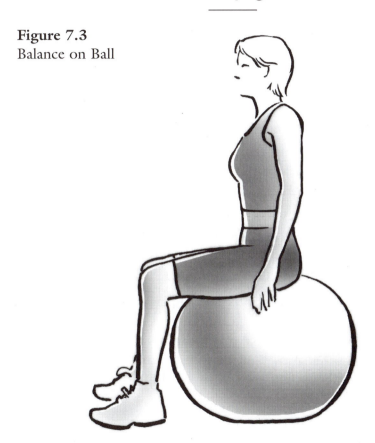

EXERCISE IV: HIP HIKERS

Hip Hikers work the abs and the quadratus lumborum muscles.

Instructions

1. Sit in correct alignment on the top of your stability ball. Your thighs should be parallel to the floor, feet flat on floor, knees over ankles. Breathe normally. Maintain neutral spine.

2. Now, perform a pelvic tilt, using your abdominal muscles to roll the pelvis backward, flattening the back. The ball will roll forward a bit. Hold briefly, then return to neutral position (not illustrated). Do 1 to 3 sets of 8–12 reps.

3. Next, from the starting position, hike your right hip up, shifting your weight into your left hip, while maintaining your balance. (The ball will move slightly in the opposite direction.) Maintain abs contraction. Then shift your weight into your right hip and raise your left hip. Do 1 to 3 sets of 8–12 reps.

Figure 7.4
Hip Hikers

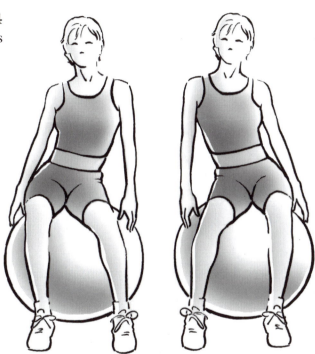

Tips and Modifications

- Use ball in an open area.

EXERCISE V: LEG EXTENSION ON BALL

Again, incorporating movement in this balance exercise works the abs harder, and also tones the legs.

Instructions

1. Sit in correct alignment on the top of your stability ball, with abs contracted. Slowly raise your right leg until it is parallel to the floor. Hold this position for 5–10 seconds, breathing normally. Release. Repeat with opposite leg. Do 1 to 3 sets of 8–12 reps.

Tips and Modifications

- If you can, raise your opposite arm into the air while extending your leg.

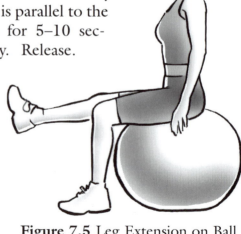

Figure 7.5 Leg Extension on Ball

EXERCISE VI: BALANCE CHALLENGE

If you're working out with a partner, this is a fun exercise for strengthening the abs and improving balance.

Instructions

1. Sit in correct alignment on the top of your stability ball, with abs contracted. (See illustration p. 105.)
2. Have a partner place her hand on your shoulder and apply constant gentle pressure so that you have to work harder to maintain your balance on the ball. (Not illustrated.)

Tips and Modifications

- Use ball in an open area.

EXERCISE VII: SWIMMING

This back strengthening exercise trains both sides of the brain to work together. It's an excellent exercise for improving neuromuscular control.

Instructions

1. Lie facedown on the floor, with legs together and arms extended overhead, resting on the floor.

2. Before initiating any movement, make sure that your hips and pubic bone are pressed into the floor and your abs are engaged. Maintain this control throughout the exercise.

3. Rotate the position of your hands 90° so that your thumbs are pointing up. This position moves the shoulders into better alignment. (Hand position not illustrated.)

4. As you inhale, raise your left arm and right leg off the floor simultaneously. Maintain abs contraction.

5. Exhale, lowering your arm and leg. Inhale, raising the right arm and left leg. Do 1 to 3 sets of 8–12 reps.

Figure 7.6 Swimming

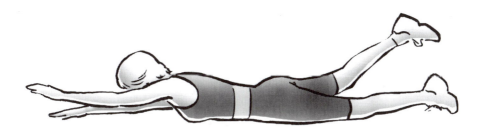

Tips and Modifications

- Keep your upper back and neck in alignment.
- For more extension in raised leg, point toes behind you.
- To increase the challenge, you can raise your chest off the floor while performing the arm and leg raises. But don't arch your neck.
- Another way to increase the challenge is to increase the pace of the exercise.

EXERCISE VIII: KNEES TO CHEST

After a strenuous back extension like the swimming exercise, you should stretch the lower back. Knees to Chest is a yoga posture that helps relieve tension in the lower back.

Instructions

1. Lie on your back with knees bent, arms at sides.

2. Slowly raise your right knee to your chest, then your left knee. Contract your transverse abdominis and press your back into the floor for support. Place your right hand on your right knee and your left hand on your left knee.

3. With an exhaling breath, gently pull your knees closer to your chest. You should feel a gentle stretch in your lower back. Inhale, releasing the stretch and allowing your knees to raise back up to a relaxing position. Repeat 8–12 times.

Figure 7.7 Knees to Chest

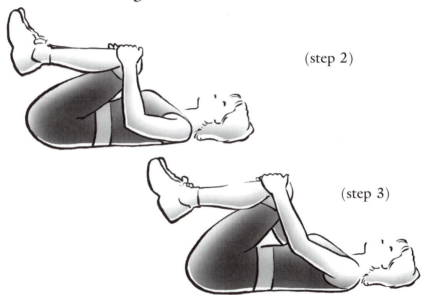

(step 2)

(step 3)

Tips and Modifications

- Practice this stretch, or other back stretches, at the end of all abs workouts.
- Spend more time stretching if needed.

8 | Workout Two: Calling All Abs

Now that you've had some practice working the deepest layer of the abs with a variety of stability exercises, you can progress to a few more traditional or "six-pack" abs exercises that work the rectus abdominis and the obliques.

The first few exercises in this group will help you work toward that "six-pack" look because they train the superficial layers of the abs, the rectus abdominis and the obliques. While the previous exercises were challenging, you will feel the burn doing most of these exercises.

The same rules apply here: Maintain neutral spine and transverse abdominis contraction throughout the exercise to protect the lower back. And use slow, controlled movements. You'll finish off this group with a functional balancing exercise and a back-strengthening exercise.

EXERCISE 1: SEATED ROTATION

This six-pack exercise works all the abdominal muscles.

Instructions

1. Sit on the floor with your knees bent. Maintaining correct posture, lean back until you feel your abs engage. Place your hands on either side of your stomach.

Figure 8.1
Seated Rotation

(step 1)

(step 2)

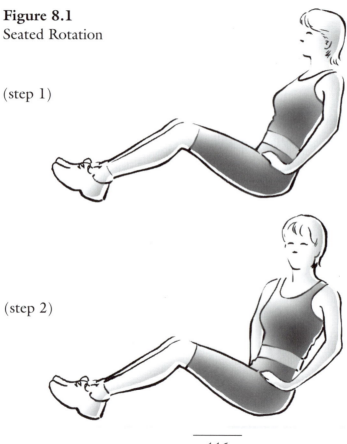

2. Using slow, controlled movements, rotate the torso to the left. Hold for a split second before returning to the center, then repeat on opposite side. Maintain correct posture and abs contraction throughout. Do 1 to 3 sets of 8–12 reps.

Tips and Modifications

• Increase the challenge by leaning back to a 45° angle in step 1.

EXERCISE II: SEATED ROTATION WITH MEDICINE BALL

By adding the challenges of weight and moving the body through a greater range of motion, you can further increase the challenge of a Seated Rotation.

Instructions

1. Sit on the floor with your knees bent, holding a 3-pound medicine ball. Maintaining correct posture, lean back until you feel your abs engage. Take a few breaths in this position.

2. With an exhaling breath, rotate the torso to the left, touching the ball on the floor to the side of the torso. Inhale as you return to center. Repeat on opposite side. Do 1 to 3 sets of 8–12 reps.

Tips and Modifications

• Maintain correct posture and constant abs contraction.

Figure 8.2 Seated Rotation with Medicine Ball

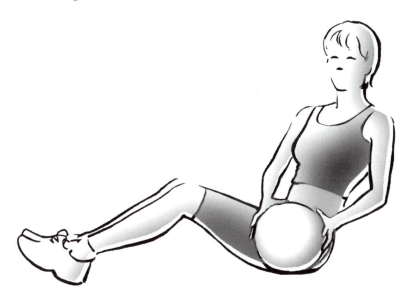

- To increase the challenge, try to straighten your arms (but don't lock the elbows) as you touch the ball to the floor.

EXERCISE III: THE PLANK

A great core strengthener, the Plank is a combination functional and stabilization exercise that provides excellent neuromuscular feedback to the brain, helping re-establish healthy muscle patterns.

Instructions

1. From a kneeling position, lean forward, placing your forearms on the floor, keeping elbows in line with shoulders. Your knees, hips, and shoulders should form a straight line.

2. Extend your legs behind you, one at a time, until you are supported both by your toes and by your forearms (similar to a push-up position).

3. Make sure that you're in correct posture and your abs are contracted. Hold pose for 10 seconds, breathing normally, but not deeply. Gradually, work up to holding the plank for 30 seconds or more.

Figure 8.3 The Plank
(step 1)

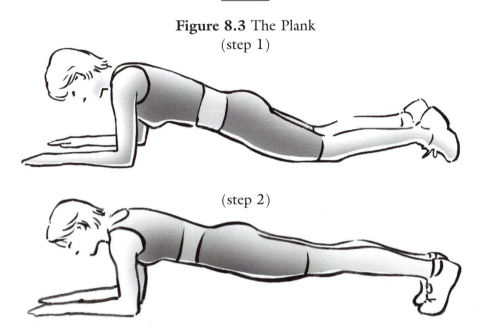

(step 2)

Tips and Modifications

- Not recommended for people with back problems.
- Follow this exercise with a back-stretching exercise like Back Stretch on page 93 or Knee to Chest on page 112.

EXERCISE IV: BALANCE WITH A MEDICINE BALL

This functional exercise works core muscles and improves balance.

Instructions

1. Stand in correct posture, holding a 3-pound medicine ball.

2. Maintaining correct posture and transverse abdominis contraction, bend your left leg so that you are balancing on your right leg.

3. In this position, move the ball around in space to challenge your balance. Extend your arms in front of you, then slowly move the ball to your right, then back to the center, and then to your left. Raise the ball over your head, then lower it to the right. Raise the ball over your head again, then lower it to the left side. Practice these movements for 2 or 3 minutes. Repeat on opposite leg.

Figure 8.4 Balance with a Medicine Ball

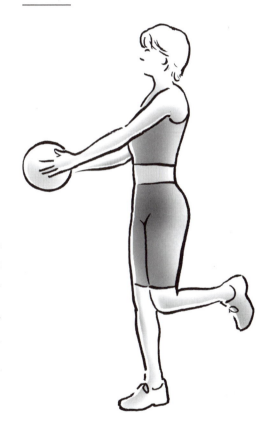

Tips and Modifications

- To increase challenge use a heavier medicine ball, but only if you can maintain form.
- It's okay to bend your supporting leg to reach more challenging positions.

EXERCISE V: REVERSE WOOD CHOP

The Reverse Wood Chop is an excellent functional exercise that trains the body for a variety of daily activities, such as lifting groceries out of your trunk or lifting your child out of his car seat.

Instructions

1. Stand in correct posture, holding a 3-pound medicine ball. Then bend your knees so that you are standing in a squat position (not a deep squat), holding the ball next to your left knee.

2. As you inhale, make one fluid movement, bringing the ball from the side of your knee to over your right shoulder (as if you were going to throw the ball over your right shoulder) as you come into a standing position. Your eyes should follow the ball as your body rotates to the side. Allow your hips to move. Maintain transverse abdominis contraction throughout movement. Repeat on opposite side. Do 1 to 3 sets of 8–12 reps.

Figure 8.5 Reverse Wood Chop

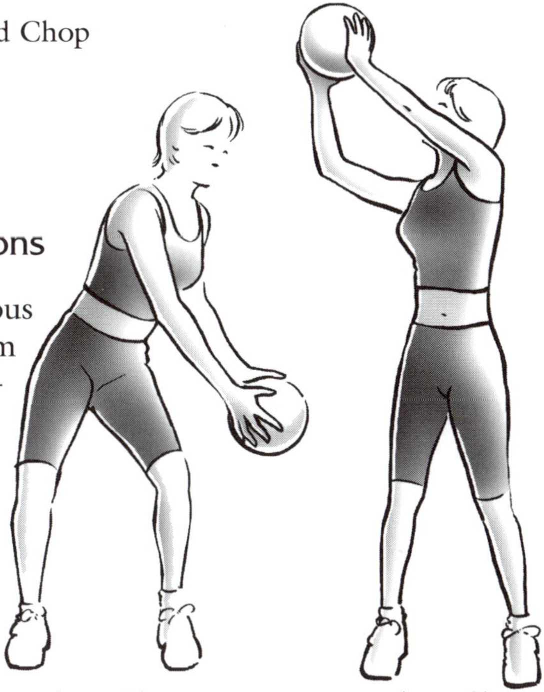

Tips and Modifications

- This is a very strenuous exercise that can harm the lower back if performed incorrectly. Make sure that you maintain your abs contraction, use a medicine ball appropriate for your skill level, and allow your hips to move with rotation.

(step 1)   (step 2)

- Follow this exercise with a back-stretching exercise like Back Stretch on page 93 or Knees to Chest on page 112.

EXERCISE VI: ALTERNATE ARM AND LEG EXTENSION

This back-strengthening exercise from Chapter 6 strengthens the erector spinae muscles that move the back and the deep multifidus muscles that support the spine. Here, you'll hold the position longer and include stretching movement in order to build greater endurance and flexibility in back muscles.

Instructions

1. Kneel on the floor on all fours. Establish correct posture (neutral spine) and contract your transverse abdominis. Breathe normally.

2. Inhale, raising your right arm in front of you and your left leg behind you, both parallel to the ground. Hold this position for 15 to 20 seconds, breathing normally. With each inhalation reach forward with your fingertips and backward with your toes (point toes) to increase the extension of your limbs and spine.

Figure 8.6 Alternate Arm and Leg Extension

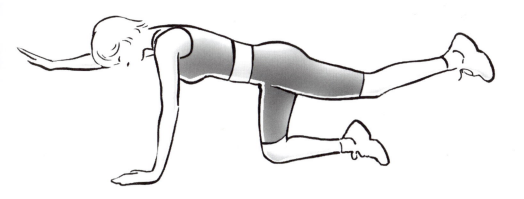

3. When you're ready to release your position, exhale as you slowly lower your arm and leg. Repeat on opposite side. Do 1 set of 8–12 reps.

Tips and Modifications

- Maintain posture and abs contraction.
- Use slow, controlled movements.
- If you can't do 8–12 reps, do as many as you can, and gradually work toward 8–12.
- Add more sets as you are able.

9 | Workout Three: The Stability Ball

Once you've mastered basic balance on the stability ball, you can practice traditional abs exercises on the ball. The instability of the ball challenges core muscles to maintain posture while you perform the movements of each exercise. Exercising on the ball is a very effective way to train the abs, giving you a "six-pack" workout. You'll find that these exercises can be quite challenging.

EXERCISE 1: MARCHING ON A BALL

Marching on a Ball, a stability exercise, takes the Dying Bug Series one step further. Again, you'll be trying to maintain neutral spine while moving your limbs, but this time with the added challenge of trying to maintain balance on your ball.

Instructions

1. Sit in correct alignment on the top of your stability ball, with abs contracted. Breathe normally.

2. Using slow, controlled movements, slowly raise your left foot off the floor several inches while raising your right arm into the air. Maintain posture, abs contraction, and balance.

3. As you lower your left foot and right arm, slowly raise your right foot off the floor several inches while raising your left arm into the air. As you did in the Swimming exercise (page 110), continue alternating these two positions. Do 1 to 3 sets of 8–12 reps.

Tips and Modifications

- The ball will move as soon as you move; try to maintain balance and form.
- To increase challenge, increase speed.
- Don't forget to breathe.

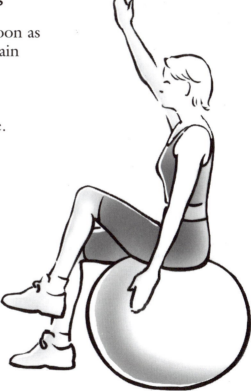

Figure 9.1
Marching on a Ball

EXERCISE II: CRUNCH ON A BALL

A great six-pack exercise, the American Council on Exercise rated the Crunch on a Ball one of the most effective at building abs strength and toning the torso.

Instructions

1. Sit in correct alignment on the top of your stability ball, with transverse abdominis contracted. Breathe normally.

2. Slowly, walk your feet out in front of you, until your lower back rests on the ball, and your thighs are parallel to the floor.

3. As you exhale, tuck your chin slightly toward your chest, and, using your abs to control your movement, slowly raise your upper body. Raise your body only until you feel tightness in your abs as your ribs move toward your pelvis. Keep your transverse abdominis contracted and your back pressed against the ball.

   You can extend your arms in front of you, rest your hands on either side of your stomach, or rest your arms, crossed, on your chest. You can also press your fingertips to the sides of your head, but don't use your hands to pull the head forward.

4. Inhale, slowly lowering your body to the ball.

5. Exhale, raising the body again, but this time rotating to the right. Inhale as you return to center, then exhale and rotate to the left as you raise your body. Do 1 to 3 sets of 8–12 reps.

Tips and Modifications

- Move your feet wider apart for better balance.
- Beginners should move the ball higher up on the back. For a greater challenge, move the ball lower on the back.

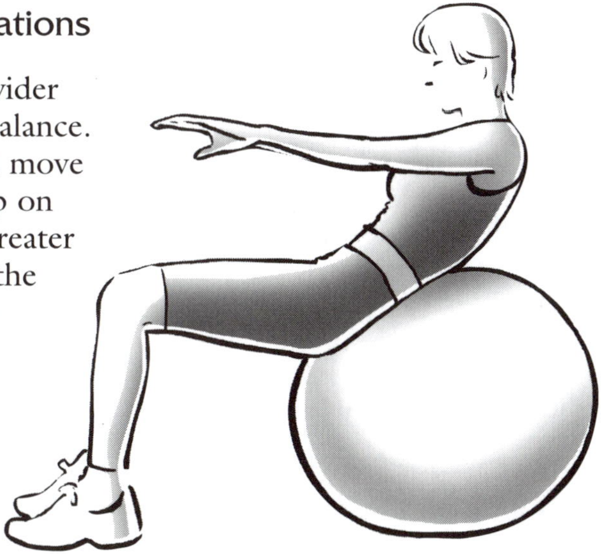

Figure 9.2
Crunch on a Ball

EXERCISE III: BRIDGING

This exercise works the abs, hips, and buttock muscles.

Instructions

1. Lie on your back with your lower legs (calves) resting on your exercise ball.

2. Inhale, engaging your abs and buttock muscles as you raise your hips off the floor. Keep your body in a straight line to maintain correct posture.

3. Hold this position for a few breaths, then slowly, using controlled movement, lower your body to the floor, unrolling the spine one vertebrae at a time, from upper to lower back. Do 1 to 3 sets of 8–12 reps.

Tips and Modifications

- To increase the challenge, begin the exercise with your heels resting on the ball.

Figure 9.3 Bridging

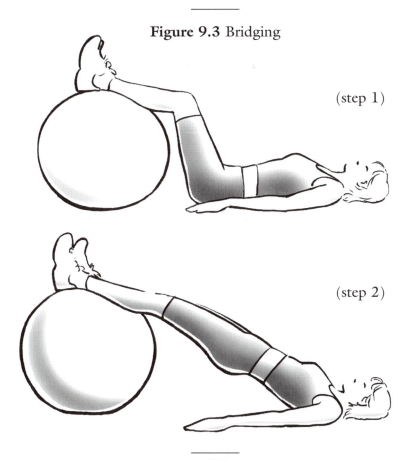

(step 1)

(step 2)

EXERCISE IV: TRUNK EXTENSION ON A BALL

Practicing Trunk Extension on a Ball strengthens back muscles for balanced core strength.

Instructions

1. From a kneeling position, rest your hips against the ball and rest your stomach and chest on top of the ball, balancing on your toes, feet hips-width apart. Place your hands on each side of the front of the ball to support your upper body.

2. As you inhale, contract your abs as you slowly raise your chest, extending your arms perpendicular to your body. Stop moving when your body forms a straight line. Use your back muscles to move, not momentum from your arms. Maintain neck alignment, eyes looking down at floor.

3. Exhale, slowly lowering your body to the ball. Do 1 to 3 sets of 8–12 reps.

Figure 9.4 Trunk Extension on a Ball

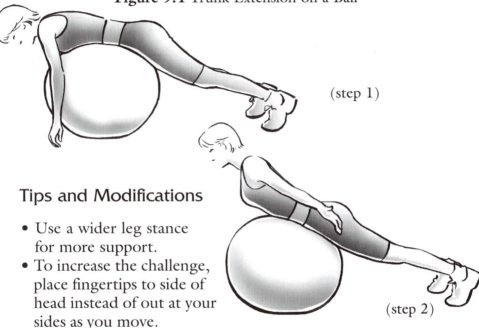

(step 1)

(step 2)

Tips and Modifications

- Use a wider leg stance for more support.
- To increase the challenge, place fingertips to side of head instead of out at your sides as you move.
- If you have back or neck problems consult your doctor before trying this exercise.
- Some people prefer exhaling with extension and inhaling with release.

EXERCISE V: ALTERNATE ARM AND LEG EXTENSION ON A BALL

Like the Alternate Arm and Leg Extension in Chapter 8, this back-strengthening exercise helps improve neuromuscular control.

Instructions

1. From a kneeling position, lean over your ball until your chest and stomach are resting on top of the ball and your hands are placed on the floor beneath your shoulders. Breathe normally.

2. Inhale, raising and extending your right arm and your left leg until they are parallel to the floor. Maintain neutral spine and transverse abdominis contraction.

3. Hold this position for 10–20 seconds, breathing normally. To release position, exhale, slowly lowering your arm and leg. Repeat with opposite arm and leg. Do 1 to 3 sets of 8–12 reps.

Figure 9.5 Alternate Arm and Leg Extension on a Ball

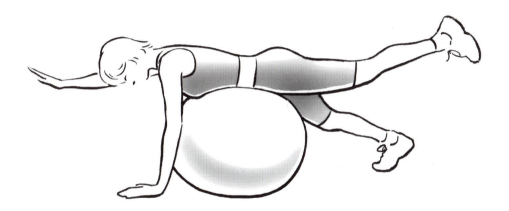

10 | Workout Four: Gym Exercises

You'll notice several of the moves in this group as traditional strengthening exercises. Maybe you didn't know these exercises had anything to do with your abs, but as you proceed you'll see how these exercises integrate core muscles with leg, buttock, arm, and shoulder muscles for overall body strength and balance.

EXERCISE I: MEDICINE BALL TWIST

Building on the Seated Rotation and Seated Rotation with a Medicine Ball in Workout Two, this combination "six-pack" and functional exercise presents an extra challenge.

Instructions

1. Lie on the floor with knees bent, feet flat on the floor, holding a 3-pound medicine ball at your chest. Take a few breaths in this position.

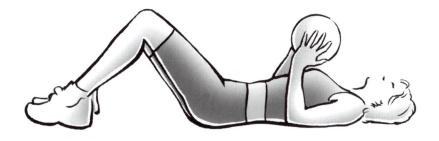

Figure 10.1 Medicine Ball Twist (step 1)

2. Exhale as you raise your torso off the floor until you feel your abs engage. Rotate to the left, touching the ball to the floor.

Figure 10.1
Medicine Ball Twist
(step 2)

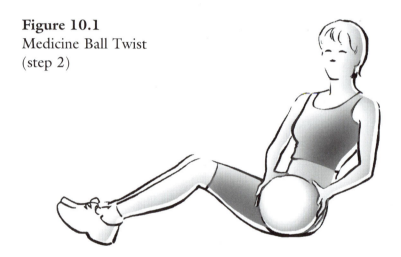

3. Inhale, slowly lowering body to the floor. Exhale, raising your torso and rotating to the right, touching the ball to the

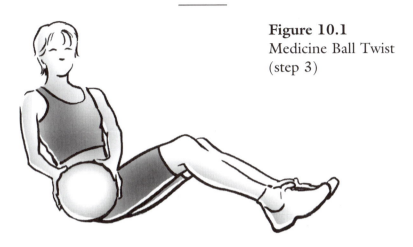

Figure 10.1
Medicine Ball Twist
(step 3)

floor. Inhale, slowly lowering body to the floor. Do 1 to 3 sets of 8–12 reps.

Tips and Modifications

- In step one, raise your body until your back forms a 60° angle with the floor. (This is approximately the position in which your abs will begin to engage.) To increase the challenge, raise your body to a 45° angle.

EXERCISE 11: BICYCLE

In a study commissioned by the American Council on Exercise, the Bicycle was rated one of the most efficient exercises for conditioning the abs. In Pilates this "six-pack" move is called the Criss Cross.

Instructions

1. Lie on your back with your fingertips at the sides of your head, legs together. Breathe normally.

2. Exhale as you pull your abs up and in toward your spine, bringing your left knee toward your chest while extending and raising your right leg to a 45° angle.

   At the same time slowly curl your head forward, chin toward chest, and raise your upper body off the floor until you feel the base of your shoulder blades against the floor. Do not pull forward with the head; raise the body using your abs. Continue breathing normally throughout the exercise.

3. Rotate your upper torso to the right, keeping your elbows wide and your chest open, reaching toward your left knee

Figure 10.2 Bicycle

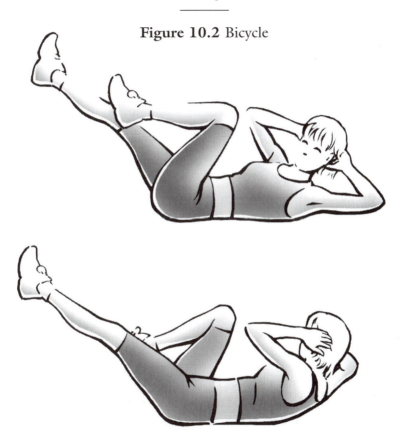

with your right shoulder as you look past your left elbow. (Touching your knee with your elbow or shoulder is not the goal.) Lowering your chin a bit toward your chest will help you as you turn your head. Do not lead the movement with elbow or shoulder, but lift and twist out of your waist.

4. Rotate your body back to the center as you switch leg positions, extending your left leg to a 45° angle and bringing your right knee toward your chest. Exhale and reach the left shoulder toward the inside of your right knee. You can lower the upper body a bit as you switch leg positions, but continue to keep the shoulder blades off the floor, abs engaged, and the backs of your hips pressed to the floor. Keep your torso as still as possible, and try not to let your body move from side to side. Do 1 to 3 sets of 8–12 reps.

Tips and Modifications

• Looking past your elbow (in the direction of the twist) when you rotate the torso will help engage the deeper layers of your abdominal muscles.

- You want to lengthen through the obliques (the sides of your torso) in this exercise, so as you twist the torso to one side, feel the extension in the opposite side of the body. Basically, as one side contracts, the other side lengthens, working the abs diagonally.
- Feel the extension in your legs as you reach the toes of your extended leg toward the opposite wall. Engaging your inner thighs and keeping your knees together will help you keep your legs in line with your hips. Keep the backs of your hips firmly planted to the floor. And don't let your extended leg drop.
- Keep chest and neck relaxed. Look straight ahead and do not let your chin fall toward your chest. As you turn to make the trunk twist, lower your chin a bit and look out past the elbow.
- Feel the top of the ab muscles, just below your sternum, engage to help rotate your upper torso. Visualize the rib cage spiraling from side to side around the spine. Twist slowly, and hold the twist as you reach back with your elbow. Exhale completely with each twist, as if you're wringing out the lungs. Remember to lift and twist at your waist; your neck and shoulders should remain relaxed.

EXERCISE III: SQUAT WITH A BALL

The squat is an excellent exercise for toning legs and buttocks. Adding a medicine ball increases the challenge of this functional strengthening exercise, forcing the abs to work a bit harder to maintain balance.

Instructions

1. Stand in correct posture, with your feet hips-width apart and your knees slightly bent, holding a 3-pound medicine ball to your chest. Breathe normally.

2. Extend your arms in front of you and lower your torso into a squat position, with your thighs parallel to the floor. Maintain neutral spine and transverse abdominis contraction. Hold this position for 5–10 seconds, breathing normally.

3. Continue to contract your core muscles. As you slowly rise to a standing position, lift the ball overhead. Return to starting position. Do 1 to 3 sets of 8–12 reps.

Figure 10.3 Squat with a Ball

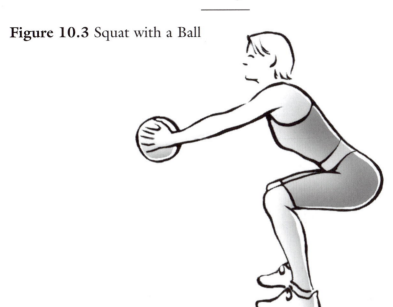

Tips and Modifications

- When raising the ball overhead, do not lock elbows but keep arms slightly bent.
- Follow this exercise with an exercise that stretches the lower back.

EXERCISE IV: LUNGE

This is another great functional exercise for incorporating core muscles with the rest of the body, with the added benefit of strengthening the lower body. Contracting your abs during a lunge helps you maintain balance and practice the lunge in correct form.

Instructions

1. Stand in correct posture, with your feet together, arms hanging at your sides. Breathe normally.

2. Maintaining neutral spine and contracting core muscles, place your hands on your hips and step backward with your left foot until you are in a lunge position, balancing on the toes and forefoot of your left foot. Your right thigh should be parallel to the floor and your left leg should form a 90° angle. Adjust your feet so that your left foot is lined up with (behind) your right foot. Hold this position for 5–10 seconds, breathing normally. Repeat on opposite side. Do 1 to 3 sets of 8–12 reps.

Figure 10.4 Lunge

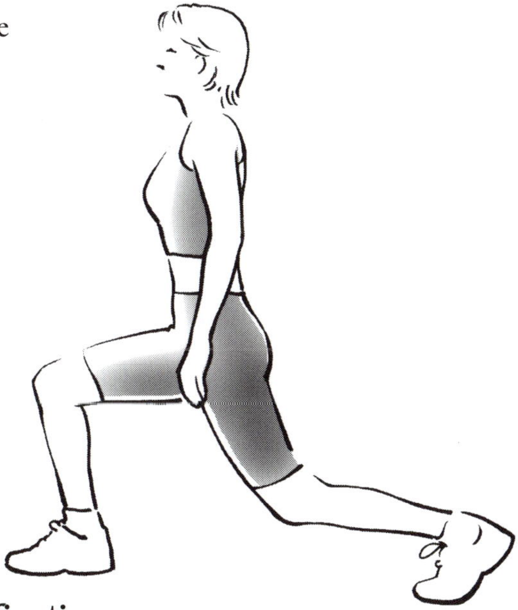

Tips and Modifications

- Further challenge the abs by lunging while holding a medicine ball.
- Follow this exercise with an exercise that stretches the lower back.

11 | Workout Five: Killer Abs

These advanced exercises are for people with a high level of fitness, whose core muscles are in great condition.

EXERCISE I: THE TABLE TOP

Like the Plank in Workout Two, the Table Top is an excellent integrative stabilization exercise that works all of the core muscles, as well as strengthens the arms and legs.

Figure 11.1 The Table Top

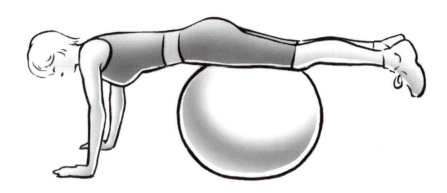

Instructions

1. From a kneeling position, lean over your ball until your chest and stomach are resting on top of the ball and your hands are placed on the floor beneath your shoulders. Breathe normally.

Figure 11.1 The Table Top (advanced version)

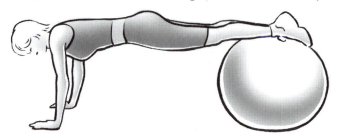

2. Maintaining neutral spine and transverse abdominis contraction, walk forward with your arms until your thighs are on the top of the ball. Hold this position for 5–10 seconds, breathing normally. Then, walk backward and return to starting position. Do 1 to 3 sets of 8–12 reps.

Tips and Modifications

- To protect your lower back, make sure that you maintain correct alignment and contract your abs throughout the exercise.
- Follow this exercise with an exercise that stretches the lower back.
- For a greater challenge, walk out until your shins are on top of the ball.

EXERCISE II: THE TABLE TOP PUSH-UP

Adding a push-up to the Table Top exercise increases the challenge to abs and back muscles to maintain optimal spinal alignment. This combination functional and stabilization move also works arm, shoulder, and chest muscles.

Instructions

1. As in the previous exercise, begin in a kneeling position. Lean over your ball until your chest and stomach are resting on top of the ball and your hands are placed on the floor beneath your shoulders. Breathe normally.

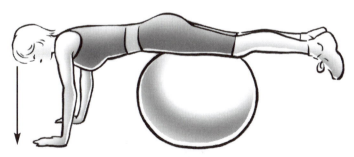

Figure 11.2 The Table Top Push-up

2. Maintaining neutral spine and transverse abdominis contraction, walk forward with your arms until your thighs are on top of the ball.

3. In this position, do 8–12 push-ups. Then, walk backward and return to starting position. Do 1 to 3 sets of 8–12 reps.

Tips and Modifications

- To protect your lower back, make sure that you maintain correct alignment and contract your abs throughout the exercise.
- Follow this exercise with an exercise that stretches the lower back.

EXERCISE III: THE SKIER

This functional exercise presents a great challenge. You'll really work core muscles trying to maintain your balance on the ball.

Instructions

1. From a kneeling position, lean over your ball until your chest and stomach are resting on top of the ball and your hands are placed on the floor beneath your shoulders. Breathe normally.

2. Maintaining neutral spine and transverse abdominis contraction, walk forward with your arms until your shins are on the top of the ball as in Table Top. Then, walk backward a bit and bend your knees so that you are balanced on the front edge of the ball in a crouching position.

3. Extend your legs, moving the ball backward, then bend your knees, returning to the crouching position. Do 1 to 3 sets of 8–12 reps.

4. If you can, press against the ball with your shins as you shift

Figure 11.3 The Skier

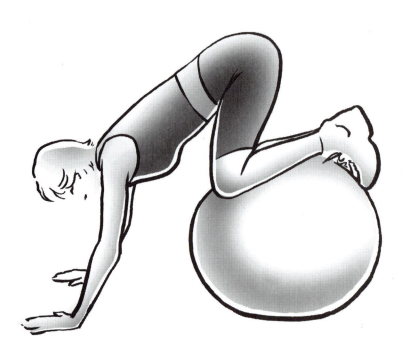

your weight into your right hip. Return to center and then shift to the left. Do 1 to 3 sets of 8–12 reps.

Tips and Modifications

- To protect your lower back, make sure that you maintain correct alignment and contract your abs throughout the exercise.
- Follow this exercise with an exercise that stretches the lower back.

EXERCISE IV: WOBBLE BOARD CHALLENGE

Trying to achieve balance on a **wobble** board is difficult enough. In this stabilization and balance exercise, the instability of the board and the weight of a medicine ball make core muscles work even harder.

Instructions

1. Stand in correct posture on a wobble board, feet hips-width apart. Try to maintain your balance as the board wobbles from side to side. Breathe normally.

2. Now try to balance on the board again, but this time, hold a 3-pound medicine ball at your chest. If you can, extend your arms and move the ball from side to side, overhead, and in other directions to challenge your balance. Try to stay on the board for several minutes.

Tips and Modifications

• Maintain neutral spine and transverse abdominis contraction.

Figure 11.4
Wobble Board Challenge

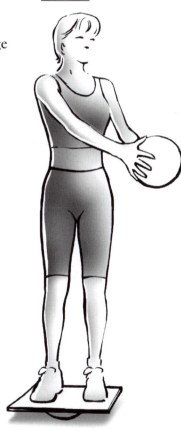

EXERCISE V: QUAD BURNER

The Quad Burner is a stabilization exercise that works core muscles, including the quadratus lumborum.

Instructions

1. Lie on your left side, with your legs together, knees bent at a 90° angle.
2. Slowly raise yourself on your left arm, with your right hand on your right hip or raised straight into the air. Hold this position for 5–10 seconds, breathing normally. Repeat on opposite side. Do 1 to 3 sets of 8–12 reps.

Tips and Modifications

- As you gain strength, you can try to do this exercise with straight legs.

Figure 11.5 Quad Burner

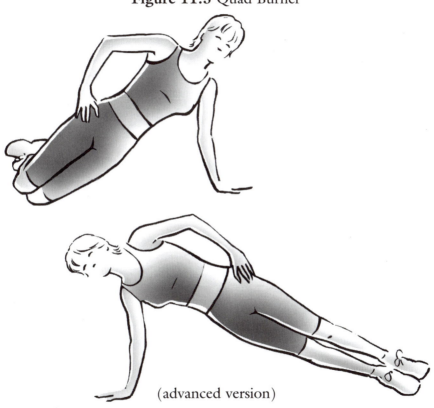

(advanced version)

EXERCISE VI: SIDE BEND WITH MEDICINE BALL

This side bend is a functional exercise that works abs and back muscles, including the quadratus lumborum.

Instructions

1. Sit in correct alignment on the top of your stability ball, with transverse abdominis contracted, holding a 3-pound medicine ball. Breathe normally.

2. Inhale, raise the ball overhead, keeping arms slightly bent.

3. Exhale, gently and slowly moving the ball 5–10 inches to the left. Imagine that you are sitting inside a tall, rectangular box, and extend the spine as if you are reaching with the ball into the top left-hand corner of that box. Hold that position for a few seconds, then inhale as you return to starting position. Repeat on opposite side. Do 1 to 3 sets of 8–12 reps.

Figure 11.6
Side Bend with Medicine Ball

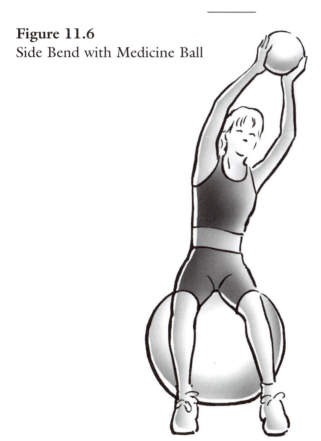

Tips and Modifications

- To protect your lower back, make sure that you maintain correct alignment and contract your abs throughout the exercise.
- Include in this workout two back-strengthening exercises such as Trunk Extension on a Ball on page 136 and Swimming on page 110.
- Follow this workout with several back stretches.
- Don't forget to breathe.

12 | Conclusion

ENDLESS ABS

With the preliminary abs exercises and five complete workouts from which to choose, you're set now for many months of abs training. Once you have established stronger core muscles, you can mix and match exercises from the different workouts, increasing the variety and number of training programs available to you.

Stay Focused

As you work on your abs, keep in mind that it takes time to feel and see change. Setting small goals and progressing slowly and gradually will help you avoid becoming overwhelmed.

Probably more than the exercises themselves, your biggest challenge will be having the discipline to do the exercises and stick with the workouts over time. Stay on track by including your abs workout in the middle of your regular fitness routine or yoga practice and by working out with a friend who can encourage you to do your exercises. Remember, it only takes five to ten minutes to do a complete abs workout.

Walk Tall

I hope that after reading this book abs exercises are no longer intimidating to you, and you feel that improving your abs is within your reach. With time, patience, and a little bit of hard work, you'll be on your way to better posture, a healthier back, and a flatter, more toned stomach.

Abspeak: A Glossary of Terms

Athletic trainer

According to the National Association of Athletic Trainers, a certified athletic trainer (ATC) is an educated and skilled professional trained to treat and rehabilitate athletic injuries. Athletic trainers work in health care settings; with high school, college, and professional athletic teams; and in health clubs.

Core muscles

Torso muscles responsible for stability and movement, primarily abs and back muscles.

GLOSSARY

Core stabilization training

A training method focused on restoring function to deepest layers of abdominal muscles that support the spine.

Crunch

An abs exercise performed on the floor, similar to a sit-up.

Functional exercises

Exercises that duplicate real-life movements, preparing the body for the various functions of daily life.

Neuromuscular control

The ability to control movements.

Neuromuscular pathways

The communication network between muscles, nerves, and the brain.

Neutral spine

The position, or range of positions, in which the spine is optimally aligned.

Optimal alignment   The spinal position best suited for pain-free, efficient movement and weight bearing.

Personal trainer   A personal trainer is a certified professional trained to design individual fitness programs to help people reach their health and fitness goals.

Proprioception   The body's awareness in space.

Repetitions   The number of times an exercise is performed. Also called "reps." For example, repeating an exercise ten times equals ten reps.

Sets   Groups of repetitions. For example, ten reps equal one set.

Six-pack exercises   Exercises that work the superficial layers of the abs, toning the stomach.

Spot reduce   A term describing a misconception that certain types of exercises can reduce fat in a specific area of the body.

Stabilization exercises   Exercises designed to retrain stabilizing muscles of abs and back.

Traditional exercises   Commonly known as conditioning exercises, including "six-pack" exercises such as the crunch.

Absources: Where to Find Fitness Equipment and Information

While researching this book I sampled exercise equipment from several different companies, including the following.

C.H.E.K. Institute
609 S. Vulcan Ave, Suite 101
Encinitas, CA 92024
800-552-8789
760-632-6360
www.chekinstitute.com
Sample products: medicine balls, stability balls, books, videos

SOURCES

Fitter International, Inc.
3050, 2600 Portland Street SE
Calgary, AB Canada, T2G 4MG
800-348-8371
403-243-6830
www.fitter1.com
Sample products: medicine balls, stability balls, wobble
  boards, books, videos

Nike
One Bowerman Drive
Beaverton, OR 97005
www.nike.com
www.niketown.com
Sample products: strength training balls (medicine balls)

The OOOF Ball Co.
454 W. Rose Tree Rd.
Media, PA 19063
800-356-6631
www.ooofball.com
Sample products: medicine balls, books, videos

Sources

Sissel
PO Box 2224
377 West 2nd St.
Sumas, WA 98295
www.sissel-online.com
Sample products: medicine balls, stability balls, books, videos

Spri Products
1600 Northwind Blvd.
Libertyville, IL 60048
800-222-7774
www.spriproducts.com
Sample products: medicine balls, exercise posters and
    books, stability balls

Thera-Band
The Hygenic Corporation
Akron, OH 44310-2575
800-321-2135
330-633-8460
www.thera-band.com
Sample products: stability balls, exercise bands and tubing

Personal Trainers

Cannonbilt Fitness Company
Peter F. Cannon
2020 13th Ave. W., #A
Seattle, WA 98119
206-283-4567
www.cannonbilt.com

Ironsmith-Fitness Doctors
1701 West 35th St.
Austin, TX 78703
512-454-4766
www.fitnessdoctors.com

performENHANCE
Christine "C. C." Cunningham
1615 Greenleaf St.
Evanston, IL 60202
847-733-0962
www.performenhance.net

SOURCES

Fitness and Health Information

The American College of Sports Medicine
401 W. Michigan St.
Indianapolis, IN 46202-3233
317-637-9200
www.acsm.org

The American Council on Exercise
4851 Paramount Dr.
San Diego, CA 92123
800-825-3636
www.acefitness.org

References

Sources consulted during research included interviews with fitness experts, books, articles, press kits and fact sheets from fitness equipment companies and the American Council on Exercise, and magazine and medical journals.

Books

Active Health and Fitness. *The Active Health & Fitness Book* (Canada: Barrie Press, 1998).

Brittenham, Greg, and Brittenham, Dean. *Stronger Abs and Back* (Champaign, Ill.: Human Kinetics, 1997).

REFERENCES

Brungardt, Kurt. *The Complete Book of Abs* (New York: Villard Books, 1993).

Brungardt, Kurt. *Essential Abs* (Emmaus, PA: Rodale Press, 2001).

Calais-Germain, Blandine. *Anatomy of Movement* (Seattle, Wash.: Eastland Press, 1993).

Chek, Paul. *Awesome Abs* (Ontario, Canada: *MuscleMag International,* 1996).

Hall, Carrie M., and Brody, Lori Thein. *Therapeutic Exercise: Moving Toward Function* (New York: Lippincott Williams & Wilkins, 1999).

Richardson, Carolyn, et al. *Therapeutic Exercise for Spinal Segmental Stabilization in Low Back Pain: Scientific Basis and Clinical Approach* (New York: Churchill Livingstone, 1998).

Articles

"Absolutely Fabulous?" Amanda Bower. *Time,* August 13, 2001.

"An Exercise Programme to Enhance Lumbar Stabilisation." Christopher M. Norris. *Orthopoedic Division Review,* November/December 1997.

References

"Application of Plyometics to the Trunk." Daniel P. O'Connor. *Athletic Therapy Today,* May 1999.

"Applying Motor Learning Principles to Exercises for the Pelvic Floor." Beate Carriére. *Advance for Physical Therapists & PT Assistants,* May 29, 2000.

"Ball-Based Education." Jolynn Tumolo. *Advance for Physical Therapists & PT Assistants,* April 12, 1999.

"Best and Worst Abdominal Exercises." www.24hourfitness.com.

"Core Body Workout." www.lifestylesport.com.

"Core Conditioning Takes Center Stage." www.ideafit.com

"Improving Neuromuscular Control Following Trunk and Lumbar Spine Injury." Julie Fritz, Annetta Haddox. *Athletic Therapy Today,* September 1998.

"Improving Proprioception and Neuromuscular Control Following Shoulder Injury." Karen Swanson. *Athletic Therapy Today,* September 1998.

"Is the AB-Doer a Don't?" Steven Loy, Alex Morice, Patrick Tssai, And William Whiting. *Ace FitnessMatters,* September/October 2001.

REFERENCES

"New Study Puts the Crunch on Ineffective Ab Exercises." Mark Anders. *Ace Fitness Matters*, June 2001.

"Physical Therapy Corner: Keeping Your Abdominal Muscles in Shape." www.nismat.org.

"Our Best Belly-Flattening Plan Ever!" Sarah Robertson. *Prevention*, March 2002.

"The New Back School Prescription: Stabilization Training Part I." Robin Robison. *SPINE: State of the Art Reviews*, vol. 5, no. 3, September 1991.

"The No-Crunch Ab Workout." www.ivillage.com.

"The Progressive Dynamic Lumbar Stabilization Program for the Treatment of Musculoskeletal Dysfunctions That Contribute to Mechanical Low Back Pain." J. Clay McDonald, K. Lee Lundgren. *Sports Chiropractic and Rehabilitation*, vol. 12, no. 2, 1988.

"The Role of Muscle Strength in Low Back Pain." Julie M. Fritz, Gregory E. Hicks, and John Mishock. *Orthopaedic Physical Therapy Clinics of North America*. 9:4, December 2000.

"What is Functional Exercise?" Paul Check, www.checkinstitute.com.

REFERENCES

Educational Materials and Instructional Videos

The Chek Institute
Thera-Band
The Ooof Ball
Spri Products
Nike
Sissel (Swiss Ball)

Notes

Chapter Two

1. Calais-Germain, Blandine. *Anatomy of Movement* (Seattle, Wash.: Eastland Press, 1993).

2. Hall, Carrie M., and Brody, Lori Thein. *Therapeutic Exercise: Moving Toward Function* (New York: Lippincott Williams & Wilkins, 1999).

3. Calais-Germain, Blandine. *Anatomy of Movement* (Seattle, Wash.: Eastland Press, 1993).

4. Calais-Germain, Blandine. *Anatomy of Movement* (Seattle, Wash.: Eastland Press, 1993).

Chapter Three

1. The "anchovy" reference comes from a comic in *Mondo Boxo,* by Roz Chast.

Index

INDEX

Index

INDEX

INDEX

Index

Index

ALSO AVAILABLE FROM WARNER BOOKS
BY ERIKA DILLMAN

THE LITTLE PILATES BOOK

Flatten your stomach, tone your thighs, and get rid of love handles—without doing crunches! A holistic exercise designed to condition body and mind, Pilates helps strengthen core muscles, improve posture, reduce lower back pain, and increase flexibility for a strong, supple body. Complete with easy-to-follow instructions and illustrations, *The Little Pilates Book* is the perfect introduction to this dynamic mat-exercise program.

THE LITTLE YOGA BOOK

Throw this book in your gym bag. Toss it in your purse, briefcase, or backpack. Use *The Little Yoga Book's* straightforward, easy-to-follow routines for midday energy boosts, to enhance other workouts, and to calm you down in the midst of chaos—anytime, anywhere. Perfect for the absolute beginner, it features simple and more advanced poses, breathing exercises, and efficient workouts. Start now and learn to enjoy more flexibility, stamina, stress reduction, and other benefits of hatha yoga.

more . . .

THE LITTLE FOOTCARE BOOK

If you've ever uttered the words "My feet are killing me!" you need this book. This fun, concise guide will teach you how to pamper your feet and enjoy the total body benefits of good foot health—even when you're always on the go. With its easy-to-follow advice, it shows you how to soothe your aching feet to reduce stress, promote relaxation, and restore energy. So take the right step with *The Little Footcare Book*.

THE LITTLE BOOK OF HEALTHY TEAS

Not your grandmother's boring brew, now tea's got a brand new bag! It helps you lift your spirits, boost your energy, and relieve cold and flu symptoms. With no fat, no calories, and half the caffeine of coffee, tea is the perfect healthy drink that relaxes, revives, and heals. Let this handy book guide you through the healing properties of this versatile tonic. Whether you prefer black, green, red, organic, or de-caffeinated tea, you'll enjoy its nourishing effects.